SHANG HAN LUN AND OTHER TRADITIONAL FORMULAS: A CLINICAL REFERENCE

SHANG HAN LUN AND OTHER TRADITIONAL FORMULAS: A CLINICAL REFERENCE

By J. Michael Moore, O.M.D.

O H A I
PRESS

美國漢方醫藥研究所出版

ORIENTAL HEALING ARTS INSTITUTE
1945 Palo Verde Ave • Suite 208 • Long Beach, California 90815

ISBN: 0-941942-42-2

First Printing: September 1995
Printed in the United States of America

Published by the Oriental Healing Arts Institute
1945 Palo Verde Avenue, Suite 208, Long Beach, California 90815

Library of Congress Cataloging-in-Publication Data
Moore, J. Michael (James Michael), 1950–
Shang han lun and other traditional formulas: a clinical reference /
by J. Michael Moore.
p. cm.
Includes bibliographical references and index.
ISBN: 0-941942-42-2

1. Medicine, Chinese--Formulae, receipts, prescriptions.
2. Herbs--Therapeutic use. I. Title.
[DNLM: 1. Medicine, Chinese Traditional. 2. Formularies. 3. Drugs, Chinese Herbal--therapeutic use. QV 740 M822s 1993]

RS131.64.M66 1993 615′.321′0951--dc20 DNLM/DLC
For Library of Congress 93-35804 CIP

ABOUT THE AUTHOR

Dr. James Michael Moore N.D., O.M.D., L.Ac., Dipl.Ac. has been studying Chinese Medicine since 1963. He received a Naturopathic Doctor degree from Pacific College, Palo Alto, California, in 1980; and a Master of Acupuncture from Occidental Institute of Chinese Studies, Miami, Florida, in 1981. He studied under private tutorship with the late Dr. Hong-yen Hsu, Oriental Healing Arts Institute, from 1985-1991. He received an Oriental Medical Doctor Degree from Southwest Acupuncture College, Santa Fe, New Mexico, in 1988.

Dr. Moore is a key figure and a very active leader in promoting the growth of Chinese medicine in the United States. He was founding president for the New Mexico Acupuncture Association, and co-founder, teacher, and assistant director for the Institute of Traditional Medicine and Southwest Acupuncture College. He helped legislate acupuncture in New Mexico, and has served as a member of the New Mexico State Board of Acupuncture. He is dean of academics for the North American Academy of Advanced Asian Medicine, and has lectured across the country.

ABOUT THIS BOOK

Traditional Chinese medicine is gaining more and more attention throughout the world. In order for a tree to bear beautiful fruit, it must have deep and strong roots. For students and practitioners of Chinese medicine to fully understand herbal prescriptions, the basic concepts found within the classics such as the *Shang Han Lun* (Treatise on Febrile Disease) and *Chin Kuei Yao Lueh* (*Jin gui yao lue*) (Prescriptions From the Golden Chamber) must be studied.

These classics are the main roots of traditional Chinese medicine. My teacher, the late Dr. Hong-yen Hsu, has stated over and over again that to truly understand traditional Chinese medicine, the classics must be studied. This book is dedicated to Dr. Hsu and his family. It has always been Dr. Hsu's dream that Chinese medicine be fully understood by the Western trained student. It is my privilege to share what he has taught me.

Ten basic disease categories are viewed from the Six Stages of Disease model which was developed more than eighteen hundred years ago by Dr. Chang Chung-ching (Zhang Zhong Jing) in his work *Shang Han Lun* (Treatise on Febrile Disease). No other Chinese medical classic rivals the *Shang Han Lun*. The treatment methods and herbs recorded therein are still being used around the world today. Eighty-seven traditional formulas are studied and arranged in such a way that the reader will have an in-depth understanding of how these prescriptions were originally used and how to use them clinically today. One-hundred sixteen individual herbs are listed herein.

Each formula is discussed in detail. First the individual herbs that make up the prescription are listed, then a general basic overview of the formula's use including: traditional function, main conformations, and major indications. Following this are quotes for the classics, whenever possible, so that a more complete understanding may be gained. This work is intended to help the reader develop a method by which any traditional formula can be organized for clinical use.

DEDICATION

This book is dedicated to the memory of Dr. Hong-yen Hsu (1917-1991), who unselfishly offered his knowledge to the world. His inspiration continues to encourage those who wish to understand herbal science and Oriental medicine. Truly, the bridge between Eastern and Western medicine has become much stronger because of his decades of research and work for all of humanity.

TABLE OF CONTENTS

CHARTS

ACKNOWLEDGMENTS

I would like to express my gratitude and thanks to my tutor and friend of six years, the late Dr. Hong-yen Hsu, Only because of him is this book possible. The following truly deserve special recognition: Dr. Daniel Hsu for his constant support and guidance, Diane Polasky, OMD, for her help in compiling information, James Varner, Ph.D., and Mei-fang Chen, MD, for their hours of editing and invaluable suggestions, and Ms. Nonie Moore, my daughter, for all her typing.

PREFACE

New practitioners of Oriental medicine are confronted with the tremendous responsibility of giving health care to their patients. One of the most commonly asked questions is: "What herbal formulas should one start with in general practice?" The formulas selected for this work have been chosen as an example that can be used for a wide range of various disorders, which a new practitioner might encounter.

For proper application it is important to have a good grasp of how and why each formula was first used by the Chinese, and how the formulas are used today. For each herbal formula, whenever possible, the Chinese classics *Shang Han Lun* (Treatise on Febrile Disease), and *Chin Kuei Yao Lueh* (*Jin Gui Yao Lue*)(Prescriptions From The Golden Chamber) are quoted so that a historical understanding of the use of each formula is brought to light. Today there are many different aspects to consider before the proper herbal formula can be prescribed. In this work a few of these will be examined so that a more systematic approach to study can be developed.

This work presents five aspects, or concepts, which are used to gain a richer and fuller understanding of how formulas can be arranged for the treatment of various diseases:

1) The model of disease pathology known as "six stages," from the *Shang Han Lun*.

2) The concepts of qi, water, and blood.

3) The basic classifications of formulas.

4) The basic conformations of formulas.

5) Western medical indications.

The model of the "six stages," in this work, is applied in various ways. From the standpoint of febrile disease, one should use the model as applied in the *Shang Han Lun*, which is discussed in detail later in this book. Although the six stages of disease was originally used for fever and chill related disorders, the basic concept can be used for almost any disease category. There are at least six different levels of disease that one should consider before an herbal formula is prescribed for treatment. Regardless of the disease or disorder one is treating, it is of utmost importance to observe a patient's overall state of health. If a patient is strong and has good wei qi (defensive energy), the body is in a state of yang (the first three levels of the six stages). This means that treatment therapies that are strong and aggressive may be used. As the disease or disorder gains strength, the body becomes weaker and there is a loss of ability to quickly utilize all of the healing responses related to wei qi. A strong or aggressive treatment may be too harsh on the body at this point, as the body is now in a state of yin (the second three levels of the six stages). This means that the ying qi (nutritive energy) of the body has become weak and cannot properly build the wei qi. A treatment must be used that can strengthen the body as well as address the various complaints.

Disease can also attack on many levels and progress in different ways. From the viewpoint of qi, water, and blood concepts, disease usually affects the body on the qi level first. If the qi is not strong enough, the overall energy of the body drops quickly and signs of water imbalance appears. Water (various fluids within the body) and blood circulate normally when the qi is strong. Soon after the water is affected by disease, the blood begins to be affected as well. Because the water yin aspect of the body cannot circulate and cool the body effectively, heat and toxins build up within the body and damage the blood. Normally, disease progresses from the qi level to the water level, and then to the blood level. However, as revealed by proper diagnosis, at times the water or blood levels may be affected even during the most acute stage of a disease. Treatment that is addressing the body on a qi level will usually have little or no effect if the disease is on a deeper level. Therefore, it is important while diagnosing any condition that the concepts of qi, water, and blood be taken into consideration before an herbal formula is prescribed.

Chinese herbal formulas are classified into twenty-four basic types, and practitioners should be able to arrive at a general idea of the basic type that a patient fits into. That is to say, before a particular formula is decided upon, one needs to have a grasp of the basic classification of the disease or disorder. For example, generally, should a sudorific formula (*jie biao ji*), interior attacking formula (*gong li ji*), sedative (*zhen qing ji*) formula, or tonic formula (*bu yi ji*) be used to treat a condition presented by a patient? Once the general classification of a disease has been established, the various conformations matching the formulas in that classification can be examined.

An herbal formula "conformation" may be one or several symptoms or signs. A patient with a common cold who also has a symptom conformation of stiff shoulders as a major complaint may require a formula like *Ge gen tang* (Pueraria Combination) as the formula of choice. A patient who is generally weak, cold, and has a sensation of fullness in the stomach may be said to have a of "weak, chill conformation of greater yin disease." The formula of choice could be *Ren shen tang* (Ginseng and Ginger Combination), which is classified as a chill dispelling formula (*qu han ji*).

Many times a patient will come in with a western diagnosis or name for an illness. This level of communication or understanding must be considered in forming an overall diagnosis. However, western names of disease only give the practitioner of Oriental healing arts an indication of one level of treatment for a condition. A patient having constipation as a major complaint in Chinese medicine, must still be considered for two major classifications of formulas:

1) Interior attacking formulas (*gong li ji*), which are basically purgatives; there are at least eleven formulas for various stages and conformations that deal with constipation in this class.

2) Dual dissolving formulas (*biao li shuang jie ji*); there are nine basic formulas in this class which are used to cause sweating for surface diseases while at the same time addressing the internal heat that causes constipation.

The intent of this work is to give the beginning practitioner of Oriental medicine, as well as those who have been in practice for some time, a system of studying and prescribing Chinese herbal formulas based on prescriptions. An effort has been made to utilize as few basic formulas as necessary so that the student may perceive the variety of ways in which these formulas can be used. Except for the more common terms, words in the pin-yin form of Chinese are italicized, and in some cases English translations are also provided. The Wade-Giles form of writing Chinese in English characters, in which many of the earlier Chinese medical texts were published, has been largely replaced by Pin-yin. In cases in which Wade-Giles usage is well known, as in the spelling of chin kuei yao lueh, Wade-Giles spelling has been retained.

Chapter 1

SIX STAGE RELATIONSHIP

According to Chinese medical theory, diseases are caused by either exogenous or endogenous factors. The exogenous factors are geography, weather, and the environment: wind, dryness, cold, fire, moisture, damp, and heat (these are referred to by several names including the six exogenous factors, six excesses, and six exterior evils). The endogenous factors are the seven emotions: joy or pleasure, anger, fear, fright, grief or sorrow, anxiety, and pensiveness or brooding. Whatever the cause, the course of a disease varies according to the individual's constitution, temperament, symptoms, nutritional status, and circulation of qi, water, and blood.

In the *Shang Han Lun,* the various stages of disease are called the "six paths": tai yang (greater yang), shao yang (lesser yang), yang ming (sunlight yang), tai yin (greater yin), shao yin (lesser yin), and jue yin (absolute yin). These stages, in turn, relate to specific acupuncture meridian pathways.

Different herbal formulas are appropriate for different stages of disease; distinctions are made in each stage according to the following differentiations:

Tai Yang

Disease at this stage attacks the upper jiao. Symptoms include headache, generalized stiffness and pain of the shoulders and neck, chills, possibly fever, and floating pulse; these are known as surface symptoms. The basic treatment in this stage is clearing the surface through medicinals that cause sweating.

Shao Yang

Diseases at this stage attack the upper jiao and middle jiao. Symptoms include a bitter taste in the mouth, dryness of the throat, vomiting, anorexia, dizziness, and a yellow tongue. Mild forms of shao yang disease can result in impaired hearing, redness of the eyes, and congestion and irritation in the chest. The basic treatment is to use harmonizing formulas; these are formulas used to treat half-external (surface) and half-internal symptoms. This conformation contraindicates both sudorific and purgative formulas.

Note: in regard to the three jiaos, when disease is moving from the exterior of the body to the interior, and from the upper jiao to the middle jiao and/or lower jiao, mixed symptoms will appear, and it will be necessary to harmonize the body for effective treatment. This is a characteristic of the shao yang stage.

Yang Ming

The middle jiao and/or lower jiao are attacked in this stage of disease, and the resulting symptoms are more serious than those in the shao yang and tai yang stages. Symptoms include a high and persistent fever, stomach and abdominal symptoms (which are often manifest in the form of abdominal fullness), anorexia, constipation, and/or diarrhea.

Tai Yin

In the tai yin stage disease attacks the middle jiao; a weak digestive system and insufficient yang qi are characteristics of this stage. Symptoms include abdominal congestion (weak fullness), vomiting, loss of appetite, severe diarrhea, abdominal pain, chest pain, warm extremities (as opposed to cold), and a slow and floating pulse.

Shao Yin

In the shao yin disease attacks the upper and lower jiaos, and frequently produces a weakened cardiovascular system and obstructed consciousness. The primary symptoms are a feeble, thin pulse and a tendency towards drowsiness. It is also important to note that symptoms in this stage have two differentiations: one is pain of the whole body, headache, chills, sometimes fever, cold extremities, and sometimes anorexia; the other is internal coldness with headache, diarrhea, anxiety, constipation, and frequent urination of clear white urine.

Jue Yin

The lower jiao is attacked in this stage of disease. Symptoms are of two types: upper body fever with lower body chills, and mixed fever and chills. Sometimes there may be only fever or only chills. Occasionally these symptoms are accompanied by flushing up of qi, hunger without desire to eat, vomiting following eating, thirst, oliguria, diarrhea with chills, and exhaustion.

Basic Essence

Shen Nong's Herbal (A.D. 25) continued the development of the concept of the four essences and their application to herbal medicine; following this concept; foods and medicines are classified into cool, warm, cold, and hot energies. Specifically, the four essences are four properties of herbs which indicate their therapeutic and physiological effects. Cold and cool, just like warm and hot, are understood to fall into the same category, but to differ in degree. This results in two categories (hot and cold) which encompass the four essences. In addition balanced, or neutral, herbs tend not to be either hot or cold; they are considered to be neutral, harmonizing, or bland herbs. Diseases whose symptoms include fever are treated with herbs which have cold or cool properties. Alternatively, chill diseases, which have symptoms of cold arms and/or legs, are treated with herbs which have hot or warm properties.

Qi, Water, and Blood Conformation

According to Chinese herbal theory, all sickness originates from poor circulation of one or more of qi, water, or blood.

Qi, as it flows through the body following the acupuncture meridian system, can become imbalanced in its circulation and cause disease. When this occurs the objective of therapy must be to harmonize the qi. Qi diseases initially affect the nervous system, and later the mind and spirit. The *Su Wen* portion of the *Nei Jing* ("The Yellow Emperor's

Classic of Internal Medicine") states that qi diseases are caused by imbalances between yin qi and yang qi. Qi diseases can be divided into mobile and static. Mobile qi disease is characterized by the uprushing movement of qi, or vitality, which causes dizziness, headaches, and flushing. Static qi disease refers to a condition of obstructed qi which accumulates in one place and causes headaches, lassitude and palpitations. If a disease affects only the qi of the body, it is not as severe as when the water balance is disturbed. If a disease has become a blood conformation, it is much more severe, and in the normal course of disease, its effect is upon the qi of the body. Qi stagnation may cause disturbance at the water level, while at a later stage the blood may be affected and/or damaged as well.

It is also important to note that excessive emotional stimulation or suppression predisposes the body to a qi imbalance which will injure the viscera and induce disease. Conformations resulting from the seven emotions, therefore, are categorized as qi diseases. Nevertheless, qi diseases often progress to affect the blood as well as the water balance of the body.

Water conformations may be caused by an imbalance in water circulation, a disturbance in metabolism, or an abnormal distribution of water, or fluid, throughout the body. The terms phlegm, mucus, and sputum all refer to the fluids in a water conformation. The most obvious water symptom is swelling of the body, or edema, but unusual urination and bowel movements, or sweating, are also considered water symptoms. In Chinese medicine the conformation of water stagnation of the stomach is "tan yin" (sputum drink), of the bronchi is "zhi yin" (branch drink), and of the kidneys or subcutaneous tissue is "yi yin" (overflow drink).

Blood conformations are caused by blood stagnation. While some cases of external blood stagnation are caused by injury, in women they are most often the result of poor circulation associated with menstruation and childbirth. Blood diseases result from malfunctions of the circulatory system and include anemia, varicose veins, hardening of the arteries, hemorrhage, irregular or abnormal menses, and problems of childbirth. Aplastic anemia, leukocytosis, and hemophilia are also associated with stagnant blood. Symptoms of stagnant blood are dizziness, headache, menstrual disorders, dark circles under the eyes, purple lips, palpitations, aching shoulders, and soreness around the waist.

Yin and Yang

In Chinese medicine yin/yang is the primary polarity from which disease and, therefore, treatment is classified. Yang disorders tend to be external or surface, acute, with fever and "strong" or "excess" in nature. Yang type patients react to disease positively, actively, progressively and warmly. Yin disorders tend to be internal, chronic in nature, with chills and generalized weakness, and deficient in nature. Yin type patients will respond to disease negatively, passively, and coolly; a yin type patient may appear relatively healthy, yet his/her illness may be difficult to cure. It is important to note that in clinical practice, complex interactions arise between yin and yang diseases, where there may be half-surface/half-internal, both chill and fever, or mixed deficiencies and excess. Moreover, various symptoms may be seen in any stage of disease and do not necessarily indicate a specific stage since the manifestations of external/internal, cold/heat, deficiency/excess vary according to the state of the individual.

Constitutional Strength

Patients are characterized as having weak, medium, or strong constitutions in regard to their health: weak is defined as having a lack of strength and muscle tone, soft pulse, slight abdominal tension, and depression; strong is characterized by good strength and muscle tone, muscle tension, and a forceful pulse; and medium is understood to have these symptoms at a medium strength, and may have some weak and some strong features at the same time.

Chapter 2

DEFINITIONS OF FORMULA CLASSIFICATION

Sudorific, or Surface Relieving, Formulas

(*Fa biao ji*)

They promote sweating, relieve muscle tension, speed eruption in measles, and eliminate surface conformations. Sudorifics act by expelling toxins accumulated on the surface of the body (skin and hair) which have not yet penetrated the interior. The sweating method is utilized to expel such toxins.

Harmonizing Formulas

(*He jie ji*)

They eliminate toxins by either coordinating the liver and spleen, or the stomach and intestines.

Dual-Dissolving, or Exterior-Interior Attacking, Formulas

(*Biao li shuang jie ji*)

They treat both the surface and the interior at the same time, or have a dissolving action in the interior as well as on the exterior at the same time.

Emetic Formulas

(*Cui tu ji*)

They cause patients to vomit sputum, undigested food, and/or toxins lodged in the throat, chest, or stomach.

Interior Attacking Formulas

(*Gong li ji*)

They attack firmness in the interior of the body, and are also called purgatives. Purgatives lubricate the intestines, promote movement in the bowel, eliminate congestion and stagnancy within the stomach and intestines, and decrease edematous swelling of the abdomen or chest.

Fever Cleansing/Fire Purging Formulas

(*Qing re xie huo ji*)

They are composed of chill and cool herbs which are used to treat fever or fire conformations. This is the type of formula used when a harmful toxin causes a fever.

Digestive Formulas

(*Xiao dao ji*)

They aid digestion and dissolve congestion--conditions are due to the malfunctioning of the spleen and stomach, impeded circulation of qi causing obstruction and distention, and movable and nonmovable tumors which have developed from accumulations of moisture, phlegm, food, and blood. Digestive formulas stimulate the circulation of qi and blood and restore normal functioning of the organs.

Summer-Heat Dispelling Formulas

(*Qing shu ji*)

They expel summer toxins and treat summer diseases. They act mainly by dispelling summer toxins or feverish diseases that occur when the earth is humid and hot. Heat dispelling formulas always include herbs that dissolve moistness, disperse surface toxin, strengthen qi, and promote salivation.

Tonic and Replenishing, or Supplementing, Formulas

(*Bu yi ji*)

They nourish and supplement inadequacies of qi, blood, yin, and yang. They act by supplementing or enriching deficiencies of qi and blood in order to adjust an over abundance of ying, thus restoring proper balance.

Chill Dispelling Formulas

(*Qu han ji*)

They are composed of warm or hot natured herbs, and are intended to dispel chill in the viscera, treat interior chill caused by yang deficiency, external chills that have invaded the interior, and yang qi which has been injured by the ingestion of inappropriate medicines.

Aromatic Inhalant Formulas

(*Kai qiao tong guan ji*)

They are composed primarily of aromatic and "penetrative" herbs, and are used to treat unconsciousness or coma due to either heat, or chill, closure.

Sedative Formulas

(*Zhen jing ji*)

They have sedating and tranquilizing effects, and reduce pain, arrest spasms, and quiet hysteria.

Astringent Formulas

(*Shou se ji*)

They are composed mainly of astringing and restraining herbs. They treat weight loss, physical debility and wasting, and exhaustion of qi, blood, and sperm. These formulas arrest sweating, coughing, excessive menstrual flow, and leukorrhea; tone the skin and muscles, and restrain prolapse; astringe the lungs and intestines; and stimulate sperm production.

Qi Regulating Formulas

(*Li qi ji*)

They balance qi and treat all qi diseases. Clinically there are many ways to treat qi disorders. These include nourishment and replenishment, discharge and guidance, purgation, expectoration, astringement, and stimulation of blood circulation. Most illnesses cannot be effectively treated without including qi herbs.

Blood Regulating Formulas

(*Li xie ji*)

They circulate the blood and treat blood diseases. Due to the number of manifestations of blood disorders, the contents of each blood formula will vary according to the action needed.

Wind Dispelling Formulas

(*Qu feng ji*)

They treat all kinds of wind disease, of which there are two major categories--those which are internal and those which are external.

Moisture Dispelling Formulas

(*Li shi ji*)

They treat body fluid (or water) illnesses. This includes both external and internal fluids as well as fluid affected by fever toxin. Diuretics increase water flow and discharge, relieve urinary stuttering, and bring about the excretion of fluids.

Moistening Formulas

(*Run cao ji*)

They utilize nourishing and moistening herbs to treat arid conformations. This includes moistening aridity with either light dispersing herbs, or with sweet and chill herbs.

Expectorant Formulas

(*Qu tan ji*)

They aid in the expulsion or elimination of excessive sputum (mucus) and saliva. Since these substances, which are water toxins, result primarily from a functional disturbance in the spleen, and secondarily the kidneys, most expectorants act as spleen-healing formulas.

Anthelmintic Formulas

(*Qu chong ji*)

They destroy parasitic worms by either dispelling them from, or killing them in, the alimentary tract.

Gyneco-Obstetric Formulas

(*Jing chan ji*)

They are specificly for women and are used to treat abnormal menstruation, excess leukorrhea, increase fertility, and problems associated with pregnancy and childbirth.

Childhood Diseases, or Pox and Measles, Formulas

(*Dou ma ji*)

They are used for a variety of childhood diseases, especially those which are of a contagious nature such as measles and pertussis, or those which attack the lungs.

Eye, or Vision Improving, Formulas

(*Ming mu ji*)

They are specificly used for the treatment of ocular diseases.

Carbuncle-Dermatosis Formulas

(*Yong yang ji*)

They cleanse fever, detoxify poisons, decrease swelling, soften hardening, and eliminate carbuncles and dermatosis caused by either internal and/or external factors. They are essentially antidotal, antiphlogistic, and fever purging in nature, and act primarily by circulating and nourishing the blood.

Note: the herbal formulas contained on the following pages have been taken from *Commonly Used Chinese Herb Formulas*, by Drs. Hong-yen and Chau-shin Hsu. Although some differ from those found in the *Shang Han Lun*, these traditional prescriptions are modifications of the *Shan Han Lun* formulas which have been adapted to modern usage.

Chapter 3

RESPIRATORY DISORDERS

The following formulas are arranged from the stronger and more aggressive to the more nutritive. The order is not absolute, but rather a basic guide to how the formulas can be arranged for treatment.

Tai Yang

During the tai yang (first) stage of respiratory disease, the following formulas should be considered:

- Ma-huang Combination
  (*Ma huang tang*)
- Pueraria Combination
  (*Ge gen tang*)
- Cinnamon Combination
  (*Gui zhi tang*)
- Pueraria and Magnolia Combination
  Ge gen tang jia xin yi zhuan xiong)
- Platycodon & Fritillaria Combination
  (*Qing fei tang*)
- Pueraria Nasal Combination
  (*Qing bi tang*)

- Minor Blue Dragon Combination
  (*Xiao qing long tang*).

Shao Yang

During the shao yang (second) stage of respiratory disease, the following formulas should be considered:

- Minor Bupleurum Combination
  (*Xiao chai hu tang*)
- Phellodendron Combination
  (*Zi yin jiang huo tang*)
- Pinellia and Magnolia Combination
  (*Ban xia hou po tang*)

Yang Ming

During the yang ming (third) stage of respiratory disease, the following formula should be considered:

- Ginseng and Gypsum Combination
  (*Bai hu jia ren shen tang*)

Yin

During the yin (tai, shao, and jue) stages--which includes the later stages of respiratory disease--the following formulas should be considered:

- Lotus Seed Combination
  (*Qing xin lian zi yin*)
- Ophiopogon Combination
  (*Mai men dong tang*)
- Lily Combination
  (*Bai hu gu jin tang*)
- Ma-huang, Aconite and Asarum Combination
  (*Ma huang fu zi xi xin tang*)
- Vitality Combination
  (*Zhen wu tang*)

Respiratory Disorder Symptoms

The following are basic disorders and indications commonly treated with the formulas in this section.

Bronchial Asthma

Symptoms: severe cough, wheezing, difficult respiration, pain in the chest, purplish fingers and lips (cyanosis), sweating, and chill of the hands and feet.

Bronchitis

Symptoms: fever (over 37°C), sore throat, cough with sputum, chest pain, and difficult respiration. During the primary stage there is watery sputum; and when the disease has become chronic, sputum becomes sticky.

Common Cold

Symptoms: mild itching in the nose, sore throat or swollen glands, and, as it progresses, fever, headache, cough, general lassitude, and muscle pain throughout the whole body.

Pneumonia

Symptoms: productive cough, hemoptysis, high fever, wheezing, chest pain, decrease of appetite, pallor, and rapid respiration. In less serious cases, mild cough and fever.

Pleuritis

Symptoms: fever, cough, pain in the chest, and difficult breathing. Pus sometimes remains in the pleural cavity due to an abscess.

Pulmonary Emphysema

Symptoms: productive cough, feeling of pressure in the chest, and difficult breathing on physical exertion. In severe cases there is abdominal weakness and a weak pulse. Although a complete cure is not possible, Chinese herbal formulas can make patients feel more comfortable.

Tuberculosis

Symptoms: productive cough, mild fever, night sweats, fatigue, wheezing, and weight loss. In the primary stage of this disease there is sometimes no obvious symptoms of illness. If the tuberculosis has been arrested, no tubercle bacillus will be found in the sputum, and the condition is not infectious.

Formulas for Respiratory Disorders

Formula	Stage	Classification	Qi, Water	Disorder	Patient Type
Ma-huang C.	tai yang	sudorific	qi	acute	strong
Pueraria C.	tai yang	sudorific	qi	acute	weak
Cinnamon C.	tai yang	sudorific	qi	acute	weak
Pueraria and Magnolia C.	tai yang	sudorific	qi	acute	medium strong
Platycodon and Fritillaria C.	tai yang	expectorant	qi	acute	medium
Pueraria Nasal C.	tai yang/ yang ming	sudorific	qi	acute	strong
Minor Blue Dragon C.	tai yang/ shao yang	sudorific	qi	acute	strong
Minor Bupleurum C.	shao yang	harmonizing	qi	acute	medium
Phellodendron C.	shao yang/ shao yin	fire purging	qi water	chronic	weak
Pinellia and Magnolia C.	shao yang/ tai yin	chi	qi water	acute	weak
Ginseng and Gypsum C.	yang ming	fire purging	qi	acute	weak
Lotus Seed C.	tai yin	fire purging	water	acute	weak
Ophiopogon C.	tai yin	moistening	qi	chronic	weak
Lily C.	tai yin	tonic	qi	acute	weak
Ma-huang, Aconite, and Asarum C.	shao yin/ tai yang	sudorific	qi	chronic	weak
Vitality C.	tai yin/ shao yin	chill dispelling	water qi	chronic	weak

Ma-huang Combination

Ma huang tang

Ma-huang	*Ephedrae Herba*	*Ma huang*	5.0
Apricot Seed	*Armeniacae Semen*	*Xing ren*	5.0
Cinnamon	*Cinnamomi Ramulus*	*Gui zhi*	4.0
Licorice	*Glycyrrhizae Radix*	*Gan cao*	1.5

This formula is used for treating common colds, headaches, fevers, general pain, and asthma in strong persons.

Functions:

Relieves exterior symptoms, promotes sweating, promotes circulation of lung qi, and suppresses asthma.

Main Conformations:

Surface-cold-firm conformation, greater yang disease caused by wind cold invasion, generalized aching, chills, and fever, but no sweating.

Major Indications:

1. Pulse; floating and tense.
2. Tongue; thin, coated white, or normal.
3. Abdomen; firm.
4. Common cold with aching and fever, but no perspiration.
5. Upper respiratory infections.
6. Rheumatoid arthritis.
7. Bronchial asthma.

References from the Classics:

Shang Han Lun, pages 9-10. "Greater yang disease with (the symptoms) of headache, fever, generalized discomfort, low back pain, aching in the joints, mild chills and gasping, but no perspiration, is treated with *Ma huang tang* (Ma-huang Combination)."

Shang Han Lun, page 11. "When greater yang disease with a floating and tense pulse, fever and generalized aching, but no perspiration, has not improved in eight or nine days, it indicates there is still a surface conformation, (If) the patient also suffers from anxiety and dizziness, and, in severe cases, epistaxis, *Ma huang tang* (Ma-huang Combination) is given.... The *shang han* condition, if associated with a floating and tense pulse, no perspiration, and nosebleed should be treated primarily with *Ma huang tang* (Ma-huang Combination)."

***Chin Kuei Yao Lueh* (Jin Gui Yao Lue),** page 116. "Ma-huang, decocted in wine in winter and water in spring, treats jaundice."

Pueraria Combination

Ge gen tang

Pueraria	*Puerariae Radix*	*Ge gen*	8.0
Ma-huang	*Ephedrae Herba*	*Ma huang*	4.0
Cinnamon	*Cinnamomi Ramulus*	*Gui zhi*	3.0
Peony	*Paeoniae Radix*	*Shao yao*	3.0
Ginger (dried)	*Zingiberis Siccatum Rhizoma*	*Gan jiang*	1.0
Jujube	*Zizyphi Fructus*	*Da zao*	4.0
Licorice	*Glycyrrhizae Radix*	*Gan cao*	2.0

This formula is used for treating febrile or afebrile common colds with chills, neck and back stiffness, inflammation, congestion, diarrhea, and muscle spasm.

Functions:

Relieves muscle aches and exterior symptoms, harmonizes nutritive (ying qi) and protective (wei qi) energies.

Main Conformations:

Yang-firm conformation, stiffness and spasms in the neck and upper back, general aching, headaches, flushingup, anhidrosis, diarrhea, and painful urination.

Major Indications:

1. Pulse; strong or floating, tense, and quick.
2. Tongue; white coated, possibly moist, and/or red.
3. Abdomen.

4. Common cold/respiratory infections with chills, and shoulder stiffness.
5. Shoulder and wrist stiffness, and neuralgia.
6. Skin diseases.

References from the Classics:

Shang Han Lun, page 9. "Greater yang disease in which there is a sensation of stiffness and heaviness in the neck and back, mild chills (anemophobia), but no perspiration, should be given *Ge gen tang* (Pueraria Combination)."

Shang Han Lun, page 9. "*Ge gen tang* (Pueraria Combination) is given to patients experiencing diarrhea as a complication of greater and sunlight yang diseases."

Chin Kuei Yao Lueh (Jin Gui Yao Lue), page 12. "Greater yang diseases with anhidrosis, oliguria, flushingup of qi towards the chest, lockjaw, and a tendency to have strong convulsions, should be treated with *Ge gen tang* (Pueraria Combination)."

Cinnamon Combination

Gui zhi tang

Cinnamon twig	*Cinnamomi Ramulus*	*Gui zhi*	4.0
Peony	*Paeoniae Radix*	*Shao yao*	4.0
Jujube	*Zizyphi Fructus*	*Da zao*	4.0
Ginger (fresh)	*Zingiberis Rhizoma*	*Sheng jiang*	4.0
Licorice	*Glycyrrhizae Radix*	*Gan cao*	2.0

This formula is used primarily during the tai yang stage. The patient will have a weak surface conformation with chills, fever with perspiration, headache, and a general loss of vitality.

Functions:

Relieve external symptoms, disperse wind, and harmonize nutritive (ying qi) and protective (wei qi) energies.

Main Conformations:

Surface weak conformation, spontaneous sweating, flushingup of qi, dry vomiting, pain under the heart, and spasm in the right abdominal rectus muscle.

Major Indications:

1. Pulse; floating and weak.
2. Tongue; thin, white coating.
3. Abdomen; weak with spasms in the right abdominal rectus muscle, and sensitivity in the hypochondrium.
4. Spontaneous sweating.
5. Common cold.
6. Eclampsia.
7. Neurasthenia.

References from the CLassics:

Shang Han Lun, pages 5-6. "The *chung feng* form of greater yang disease accompanied by a floating pulse (superficial palpation), or weak pulse (deep palpation), mild or severe chills, persistent fever, nasal irritation and congestion, and nausea, should be treated primarily with *Gui zhi tang* (Cinnamon Combination)."

Shang Han Lun, page 6. "*Gui zhi tang* (Cinnamon Combination) should be given (to patients with) greater yang disease who have headaches, fever, perspiration, and mild chills (anemophobia). (It) is given for cases of greater yang disease that have been treated with the purgation method, but have upward congestion from the chest to the pharynx."

Shang Han Lun, page 7. "If, after the first administration of *Gui zhi tang* (Cinnamon Combination) for greater yang disease, there is continued distress instead of recovery, acupuncture should be performed at points (*feng zhi*, GB- 20) and *feng fu* (GV-16) in order to disperse the *qi*. Then *Gui zhi tang* is given to effect a cure.

In the presence of continued profuse sweating and a large pulse without thirst after one administration of *Gui zhi tang*, (Cinnamon Combination), a second dose should be given as recommended in the preceding paragraph. If improvement is not complete and there are mild, daily recurring malaria-like symptoms, but no perspiration, recovery will be delayed until perspiration occurs. *Gui zhi er ma huang yi tang* (Ma-huang and Double Cinnamon Combination) is recommended under these circumstances."

Shang Han Lun, page 8. "Those cases treated with (*Gui zhi tang* (Cinnamon Combination) and the purgation method, in which there are still headaches, stiffness of the neck, persistent fever without perspiration, fullness beneath the heart with mild aching, and dysuria, should be given *Gui zhi zhu gui jia fu ling bai zhu tang* (Hoelen, Atractylodes, and Peony Combination). Cases of the *shang han* condition that exhibit a floating pulse, spontaneous perspiration, polyuria, distress, mild chills, and foot spasms, should not be treated with *Gui zhi tang* (Cinnamon Combination) as it would cause more severe chills in the limbs, dryness of the pharynx, continued distress, and vomiting."

Shang Han Lun, page 10. "When the outside conformation of the greater yang disease is not relieved by the sweating method, as evidenced by a floating and weak pulse, *Gui zhi tang* (Cinnamon Combination) may be given."

Shang Han Lun, page 11. "When the surface conformation of *Gui zhi tang* (Cinnamon Combination) of greater yang disease is not relieved, *Gui zhi tang* (Cinnamon Combination) is recommended rather than the purgation method."

Shang Han Lun, page 12. "The patient with generalized aching, and a sinking and slow pulse, should be treated, after inducing perspiration, mainly with *Gui zhi tang* (Cinnamon Combination), to which has been added one liang (31.25 grams) each of peony and ginger, and three liang (93.75 grams) of ginseng."

"The patient who gasps after perspiring should not be given additional *Gui zhi tang* (Cinnamon Combination). Those without a severe fever who are subject to gasping after perspiring may be given *Ma xing gan shi tang* (Apricot Seed and Ma-huang Combination)."

Shang Han Lun, page 45-46. "Both the sweating method and *Gui zhi tang* (Cinnamon Combination), a formula for the surface fever conformation of greater yang disease, are recommended for patients with greater yin disease who have diarrhea, abdominal congestion, and a floating pulse (a symptom of surface fever)."

Shang Han Lun, page 56. "Cases with a combination of diarrhea, abdominal fullness due to interior weakness and chills, generalized aching as a result of surface fever, should be treated first for the interior chills by warming with *Si ni tang* (Aconite and G.L. Combination), and then for the surface (fever) by purging with *Gui zhi tang* (Cinnamon Combination)."

Shang Han Lun, page 59. "*Xiao chai hu tang* (Minor Bupleurum Combination) is recommended for patients who have recovered from a shang han condition, but who are having relapses of fever. If the patient has a floating pulse (a conformation of "surface" disease), a mild sweating agent such as *Gui zhi tang* (Cinnamon Combination) is recommended. A mild purgation agent such as *Tiao wei cheng qi tang* (Rhubarb and Mirabilitum Combination) is given to patients with a sinking solid pulse (inside firmness) in post-illness conditions."

Chin Kuei Yao Lueh (Jin Gui Yao Lue), page 12. "Greater yang disease with anhidrosis, oliguria, flushingup of qi towards the chest, lockjaw, and a tendency to have strong convulsions...can be treated with *Gui zhi tang* (Cinnamon Combination)."

Chin Kuei Yao Lueh (Jin Gui Yao Lue), page 70. "Chill colic with abdominal aching, adverse chills, cold and numb extremities, and generalized aching unresponsive to moxibustion acupuncture and other drugs, should be treated with *Wu tou gui zhi tang* (Wu-tou and Cinnamon Combination)."

Chin Kuei Yao Lueh (Jin Gui Yao Lue), page 129. "A patient with diarrhea, distention of the abdomen, and generalized aching, should be treated by first warming the interior (with *Si ni tang* (Aconite, Ginger, and Licorice C.)) before attacking the surface symptoms with (*Gui zhi tang* (Cinnamon Combination)."

Chin Kuei Yao Lueh (Jin Gui Yao Lue), page 140. "When a pregnant woman has an otherwise normal pulse that feels thin and weak on the *zhi* site, thirst, and a loss of appetite, but no chills and fever, she should take *Gui zhi tang* (Cinnamon Combination). These symptoms usually appear during the first 60 days of pregnancy."

Chin Kuei Yao Lueh (Jin Gui Yao Lue), pages 147-148. "A woman who has been suffering from evil wind without relief for 20 to 30 days after delivery--mild headache, chillphobia, frequent fever, depression beneath the heart, dry heaves, and excessive perspiration--has a *Gui zhi tang* (Cinnamon Combination) conformation. Despite the length of suffering, this formula may be given."

Pueraria and Magnolia Combination

Ge gen tang jia xin yi chuan xiong

Ma-huang	*Ephedrae Herba*	*Ma huang*	4.0
Cinnamon twig	*Cinnamomi Ramulus*	*Gui zhi*	2.0
Peony	*Paeoniae Radix*	*Shao yao*	2.0
Licorice	*Glycyrrhizae Radix*	*Gan cao*	2.0
Pueraria	*Purariae Radix*	*Ge gen*	4.0
Jujube	*Zizyphi Fructus*	*Da zao*	3.0
Cnidium	*Cnidii Rhizoma (Ligustici Rhizoma)*	*Chuan xiong*	3.0
Magnolia flower	*Magnoliae Liliflora Flos*	*Xin yi*	3.0
Ginger	*Zingiberis Rhizoma*	*Sheng jiang*	1.0

This formula acts as a sedative and antispasmodic; it is good for symptoms of headache, neck, back, or shoulder stiffness, chills, oliguria, stuffy nose with sneezing, sore throat, toothache, and convulsions.

Functions:

Relieves muscle aches and exterior symptoms, promotes blood circulation, and alleviates pain.

Main Conformations:

Neck, shoulder or upper back stiffness, anhidrosis, stuffy nose, oliguria, and severe chills.

Major Indications:

1. Pulse; floating and excess.
2. Tongue; coated with white fur.
3. Abdomen: normal.
4. Colds that are now involving the lungs; i.e. bronchitis.

5. Earache.
6. Rheumatic pain and neuralgia.
7. Acute colitis.
8. Toothache.

Platycodon & Fritillaria Combination

Qing fei tang

Scute	*Scutellariae Radix*	*Huang qin*	2.0
Platycodon	*Platycodi Radix*	*Jie geng*	2.0
Morus Bark	*Mori radicis Cortex*	*Sang bai pi*	2.0
Apricot Seed	*Armeniacae Semen*	*Xing ren*	2.0
Gardenia	*Gardeniae Fructus*	*Zhi zi*	2.0
Asparagus	*Asparagi Radix*	*Tian men dong*	2.0
Fritillaria	*Fritillariae Bulbus*	*Bei mu*	2.0
Citrus	*Citri Leiocarpae Exocarpium*	*Chen pi*	2.0
Jujube	*Zizyphi Fructus*	*Da zao*	3.0
Bamboo (shavings)	*Bambusae Caulis Et Taeniis*	*Zhu ru*	2.0
Hoelen	*Poria*	*Fu ling*	3.0
Tang-kuei	*Angelicae Radix*	*Dang gui*	3.0
Ophiopogon	*Ophiopogonis Tuber*	*Mai men dong*	3.0
Schizandra	*Schizandrae Fructus*	*Wu wei zi*	0.5
Ginger (fresh)	*Zingiberis Rhizoma*	*Sheng jiang*	0.5
Licorice	*Glycyrrhizae Radix*	*Gan cao*	1.0

This formula, which is both cooling and nourishing, is used as an expectorant to treat chronic respiratory disease in weak persons, and especially when there is internal heat resulting in deep sputum and irritation.

Functions:

Clears and moistens lungs, dissolves phlegm, and arrests cough.

Main Conformations:

Sore throat, severe cough, flushingup of qi, thick sputum, and chronic fever.

Major Indications:

1. Pulse; rapid and weak.
2. Tongue; red with no coating, or with thick yellow fur; possibly may have red dots near the tip.
3. Abdomen: N/A.
4. Chronic respiratory disorders.
5. Fever.
6. Severe cough.

Pueraria Nasal Combination

Qing bi tang

Pueraria	*Purariae Radix*	*Ge gen*	6.0
Cnidium	*Cnidii Rhizoma (Ligustici Rhizoma)*	*Chuan xiong*	1.5
Ma-huang	*Ephedrae Herba*	*Ma huang*	3.0
Rhubarb	*Rhei Rhizoma*	*Da huang*	1.5
Cinnamon Bark	*Cinnamomi Cortex*	*Gui pi*	2.5
Licorice	*Glycyrrhizae Radix*	*Gan cao*	1.0
Peony	*Paeoniae Radix*	*Shao yao*	3.0
Coix	*Coicis Semen*	*Yi yi ren*	5.0
Ginger	*Zingiberis Rhizoma*	*Sheng jiang*	1.5
Platycodon	*Platycodi Radix*	*Jie geng*	4.5
Gypsum	*Gypsum Fibrosum*	*Shi gao*	2.0
Jujube	*Zizyphi Fructus*	*Da zao*	2.0
Magnolia Flower	*Magnoliae Liliflora Flos*	*Xin yi*	4.0

This formula is used to treat wind chill disorders with symptoms of nasal discharge and stuffiness, sneezing, chillphobia, fatigue, headache, nose and throat itching, and body ache.

Functions:

Clears nasal passages, opens frontal cavities, and improves energy and mental state.

Main Conformations:

Headache, stiff neck and shoulders, nose suppuration, and rhinitis.

Major Indications:

1. Pulse; floating and strong, or moderate.
2. Tongue; thin or moderate white fur.
3. Abdomen; N/A.
4. Common cold.
5. Stiff neck and shoulders.
6. Acute rhinitis.

Minor Blue Dragon Combination

Xiao qing long tang

Pinellia	*Pinellia Tuber*	*Ban xia*	6.0
Ma-huang	*Ephedrae Herba*	*Ma huang*	3.0
Peony	*Paeoniae Radix*	*Shao yao*	3.0
Licorice	*Glycyrrhizae Radix*	*Gan cao*	3.0
Cinnamon Twigs	*Cinnamomi Ramulus*	*Gui zhi*	3.0
Asarum	*Asari Herba Cum Radice*	*Xi xin*	3.0
Schizandra	*Schizandrae Fructus*	*Wu wei zi*	3.0
Ginger (dried)	*Zingiberis Siccatum Rhizoma*	*Gan jiang*	3.0

This formula is used for both acute surface conditions and chronic disorders, both of which require a warming action. The formula is safe to use over a long term with average-weak type patients. It is used in upper respiratory disorders where there is cough with fever, chills, dyspnea, and upflushing. It is the first choice in Japan for treating asthma in children, but is contraindicated when there are night sweats.

Functions:

Relieves external conformations, warms the body, and prevents coughing and asthma.

Main Conformations:

Dry vomit, frothy or watery sputum, asthmatic cough, upflushing, facial edema, lower abdominal fullness, and decreased urine.

Major Indications:

1. Pulse; floating, thin, and quick.
2. Tongue; moist and glossy, or with a white, thick coat.
3. Abdomen; full with water toxins.
4. Upper respiratory disorders with watery sputum and coughing.
5. Asthma.
6. Pulmonary asthma.
7. Allergies.
8. Overall damp symptoms.
9. Edema or edematous disorders.

References from the Classics:

Shang Han Lun, page 10. "*Xiao qing long tang* (Minor Blue Dragon Combination) is indicated for *shang han* conditions when the surface symptoms--water (fluid) beneath the heart, retching, fever, cough, thirst, diarrhea, hiccoughs, dysuria, fullness of the lower abdomen, and gasping--are not relieved."

Shang Han Lun, page 10. "*Shang han* conditions with water (fluid) beneath the heart resulting in coughing, wild gasping, and fever without thirst, should be treated primarily with *Xiao qing long tang* (Minor Blue Dragon Combination)."

Chin Kuei Yao Lueh (Jin Gui Yao Lue), page 84. *Xiao qing long tang* (Minor Blue Dragon Combination) treats patients with overflowing stagnancy by inducing sweating."

Chin Kuei Yao Lueh (Jin Gui Yao Lue), page 89. "Coughing and gasping that prevents one from lying down should be treated with *Xiao qing long tang* (Minor Blue Dragon Combination)."

Chin Kuei Yao Lueh (Jin Gui Yao Lue), page 153. "A slobbering woman who undergoes purgation, and has only an obstruction beneath the heart to be treated should first be given *Xiao qing long tang* (Minor Blue Dragon Combination)."

Minor Bupleurum Combination

Xiao chai hu tang

Bupleurum	*Bupleuri Radix*	*Chai hu*	7.0
Scute	*Scutellariae Radix*	*Huang qin*	3.0
Pinellia	*Pinellia Tuber*	*Ban xia*	5.0
Ginseng	*Ginseng Radix*	*Ren shen*	3.0
Jujube	*Zizyphi Fructus*	*Da zao*	3.0
Licorice	*Glycyrrhizae Radix*	*Gan cao*	2.0
Ginger (fresh)	*Zingiberis Rhizoma*	*Sheng jiang*	4.0

Minor Bupleurum Combination is a harmonizing formula used for persons of average constitution experiencing symptoms associated with shao yang disease. The disease affects both the internal and external parts of the body, and will manifest primarily in the liver/gallbladder energy of the body. Symptoms may include chest distention, hardness beneath the heart, pain beneath the ribs and liver, loss of appetite, stress, vomiting, abdominal pain, bitter taste in the mouth, and recurrent fever and chills.

Functions:

Soothes liver, cleanses gallbladder, and treats half-exterior/half-interior conformations.

Main Conformations:

Half-surface/half-interior conformation, headache, deafness, bitter taste in mouth, tongue coated with white fur, loss of appetite, alternating chills and fever, chest pain, thoracocostal distress, abdominal pain, and rigidity of the neck.

Major Indications:

1. Pulse; wiry/tight, and either thin or quick.
2. Tongue; coated with white fur.
3. Abdomen; fullness and tightness in the upper abdomen and under the ribs, and palpitations below the heart in the hypochondric area.
4. Common cold and upper respiratory infections with lingering fever and viscid sputum.

5. Liver and gallbladder disorders.
6. Thoracocostal and hypochondric fullness/obstruction.
7. Gastric disorders.
8. Infections of lymph, breasts, tonsils, lungs, uterus, and so forth.
9. Mental instability in children.

References from the Classics:

Shang Han Lun, page 16. "If the *shang han* condition persists for five to six days with alternating chills and fever, distress and fullness in the chest and ribs, silence with loss of appetite, disturbances in the heart with a tendency to vomit or disturbances in the chest without vomiting, thirst, abdominal aching, obstruction and stiffness beneath the ribs; or palpitations beneath the heart, dysuria, adypsia, mild generalized fever, or cough, *Xiao chai hu tang* (Minor Bupleurum Combination) is indicated."

"For shang han conditions that have persisted for four to five days with somatic fever, severe chills, stiffness of the neck, fullness beneath the ribs, warm limbs, and thirst, *Xiao chai hu tang* (Minor Bupleurum Combination) is indicated."

Shang Han Lun, page 17. "Patients with a shang han condition with an obstructed, rough pulse on superficial palpation and a tense pulse on deep touch will have an acute abdominal ache and should first take *Xiao jian zhong tang* (Minor Cinnamon and Peony Combination). If recovery is not complete, *Xiao chai hu tang* (Minor Bupleurum Combination) should be taken."

"Sometimes greater yang disease persists for more than ten days and moves slowly into the lesser yang stage. If it has been mistakenly treated with two or three purgations under the assumption that the disease has shifted to the sunlight yang stage, and four or five days later it still exhibits *Xiao chai hu tang zhen* (conformation of the Minor Bupleurum Combination), it should now be treated with *Xiao chai hu tang* (Minor Bupleurum Combination). In cases of severe vomiting after taking this combination, plus unrelieved stagnancy beneath the heart and distress in the chest, treatment with *Da chai hu tang* (Major Bupleurum Combination) may result in recovery after an episode of diarrhea."

Shang Han Lun, page 17-18. "If the *shang han* condition has persisted for about thirteen days, with fullness between the chest and ribs, vomiting lesser yang and *Chai hu tang* zhen (conformation of Bupleurum Combinations), tidal fever at sunset sunlight yang and *Cheng qi tang zhen* (conformation of Rhubarb Combination) and mild diarrhea, *Xiao chai hu tang* (Minor Bupleurum Combination) is recommended to relieve the surface symptoms followed by *Diao wei zheng qi tang* (Bupleurum and Mirabilitum Combination)."

Shang Han Lun, page 22. "Women with *zhong feng* conditions lasting seven to eight days, lingering chills and fever occurring at regular intervals (malaria-like symptoms), and amenorrhea and stagnancy of the blood, should be treated primarily with *Xiao chai hu tang* (Minor Bupleurum Combination)."

Shang Han Lun, page 23. "*Shang han* conditions lasting five or six days with perspiration in the head area, mild chills, coldness of the hands and feet (two symptoms of lesser yin disease), congestion beneath the heart, loss of appetite (evidence of lesser yang disease), hard stools, and a small pulse, may be treated with *Xiao chai hu tang* (Minor Bupleurum Combination). Recovery will occur when the bowel movements return to normal, an effect of Minor Bupleurum Combination."

Shang Han Lun, page 38-39. "Sunlight yang disease, when present in combination with lesser yang disease, may exhibit hardness and congestion beneath the ribs, constipation (stagnancy in the lower jiao), vomiting (disharmony in the middle jiao), and white coating on the tongue (stagnancy in the upper jiao). *Xiao chai hu tang* (Minor Bupleurum Combination) is given to treat the upper jiao. When the upper jiao is normalized, the body fluids will then descend and circulate in the triple jiao, and the stomach will be harmonized. The problem is usually resolved following marked perspiration."

Shang Han Lun, page 39. "The *zhong feng* condition of sunlight yang disease is a combination of the three yang diseases. The symptoms are tension (lesser yang), floating (greater yang) and large (sunlight yang) pulse, rapid respiration, abdominal congestion (sunlight yang conformation), pain beneath the ribs and aching over the pericardium (lesser yang conformation), difficulty when pressure is applied to the abdomen, dryness of the nose, lack of perspiration (greater yang conformation), drowsiness, yellowish discoloration of the face and body (jaundice), difficulty in urination, tidal fever, frequent hiccoughs, and swelling around the ears (lesser yang conformation). If the swelling recedes following acupuncture, but the outside symptoms linger for more than ten days with the floating pulse as before, then *Xiao chai hu tang* (Minor Bupleurum Combination) should be administered."

Shang Han Lun, page 44. "For patients with unrelieved manifestations of greater yang disease complicated by symptoms of lesser yang disease including hardness and congestion beneath the ribs, retching, loss of appetite, alternating chills and fever, and a sinking and tight pulse, *Xiao chai hu tang* (Minor Bupleurum Combination) is recommended if vomiting or purgation methods have not been applied. If moxibustion, vomiting, or sweating methods have been used and there is delirium, it is of ominous import and indicates that the case has been mistreated. Now it is too late to institute the *chai hu qi* (bupleurum-containing formulas) as treatment."

Shang Han Lun, page 59. "*Xiao chai hu tang* (Minor Bupleurum Combination) is recommended for patients who have recovered from *shang han* conditions, but have relapses of fever."

Chin Kuei Yao Lueh (Jin Gui Yao Lue), page 116. "*Xiao chai hu tang* (Minor Bupleurum Combination) treats conditions of jaundice with vomiting, and abdominal aching."

Chin Kuei Yao Lueh (Jin Gui Yao Lue), page 124. "A patient with vomiting and fever should be treated primarily with *Xiao chai hu tang* (Minor Bupleurum Combination)."

Chin Kuei Yao Lueh (Jin Gui Yao Lue), page 146. "When a puerperal woman has depressive dizziness, a minute and weak pulse, vomits and has no appetite, passes hard stools, and perspires on the head only, it is due to blood weakness and its consequent flushing of yang. The flushing definitely results in dizziness, and the patient perspires profusely before the dizziness is relieved. Blood weakness and chills in the lower jiao lead to flushing of solitary yang and consequent sweating on the head. A puerperal woman needs to perspire because exhaustion of yin and blood weakness lead to excessive yang. Sweating restores the balance of yin and yang. *Xiao chai hu tang* (Minor Bupleurum Combination) treats a conformation of hard stools, vomiting, and loss of appetite."

Chin Kuei Yao Lueh (Jin Gui Yao Lue), page 149. "When a puerperal woman has contracted wind evil because of exposure of her lower body during labor, and thus has limb distress, annoying fever and a headache, she can be given *Xiao chai hu tang* (Minor Bupleurum Combination)."

Chin Kuei Yao Lueh (Jin Gui Yao Lue), page 151. "A woman with contraction of winds (i.e., heat in the liver) will have alternating seizures of chills and fever at fixed hours. The seizures last for seven to eight days and interrupt the menses. The fever, upon invading the womb, causes the blood to stagnate and produce malaria-like symptoms. The woman requires treatment with *Xiao chai hu tang* (Bupleurum Combination)."

Phellodendron Combination

Zi yin jiang huo tang

Tang-kuei	*Angelicae Radix*	*Dang gui*	2.5
Peony (red)	*Paeoniae Rubra Radix*	*Chi shao*	2.5
Rehmannia (raw)	*Rehmanniae Radix*	*Sheng di huang*	2.5
Asparagus	*Asparagi Radix*	*Tian men dong*	2.5
Ophiopogon	*Ophiopogonis Tuber*	*Mai men tong*	2.5
Citrus	*Citri Leiocarpae Exocarpium*	*Chen pi*	2.5
Atractylodes (white)	*Atractylodis rhizoma*	*Bai shu*	3.0
Anemarrhena	*Anemarrhenae Rhizoma*	*Zhi mu*	1.5
Licorice	*Glycyrrhizae Radix*	*Gan cao*	1.5
Phellodendron	*Phellodendri Cortex*	*Huang bo*	1.5

This fire purging formula is used in deficient lung yin conditions, but is more aggressive than *Mai men dong tong* (Ophiopogon Combination), so the patient should be of a stronger constitution. Symptoms include fever and coughing associated with depletion of fluids, yin weakness, and general depletion.

Functions:

Clears heat and fire, and nourishes yin.

Main Conformations:

Yin weakness with fire agitation, dry cough, thick sticky sputum, fever, anhidrosis, and pale, dark and withered skin

Major Indications:

1. Pulse; weak, and rapid; and in more severe cases, thready.
2. Tongue; red body, and possibly a dry-yellow-to-brown coat.
3. Abdomen; hard.
4. Respiratory disorders.
5. Constipation.
6. Dry cough.
7. Kidney disorders.
8. Diabetes, and nocturnal emissions

Pinellia and Magnolia Combination

Ban xia hou po tang

Pinellia	*Pinellia Tuber*	*Ban xia*	6.0
Magnolia Bark	*Magnoliae Officinalis Cortex*	*Hou pu*	3.0
Hoelen	*Poria*	*Fu ling*	5.0
Ginger (fresh)	*Zingiberis Rhizoma*	*Sheng jiang*	4.0
Perilla Leaves	*Perillae Folium*	*Zi su ye*	2.0

This formula is used for an average-weak person with stomach and chest symptoms manifesting as stagnant qi. This includes respiratory disorders associated with stress and emotional instability, decreased abdominal and general muscle tonis, and delicate constitution.

Functions:

Regulates qi, disperses stagnancy, subdues flushingup, and dispels stagnant phlegm and water.

Main Conformations:

Facial edema, glassy eyes, facial anemia, sensation of something stuck in the throat (plum pit qi, globus hystericus), weak gastrointestinal tract with water stagnation, and decreased urine.

Major Indications:

1. Pulse; floating and weak, or submerged and thin.
2. Tongue; pale or purple.
3. Abdomen; weakness with wate sloshing (stagnant water in stomach).
4. Mental instability, nervousness, and insomnia.
5. Palpitations.
6. Gastrointestinal weakness.
7. Fatigue.
8. Flushingup.
9. Cough, and asthma.
10. Edema.
11. Toxemia during pregnancy.

References from the Classics:

Chin Kuei Yao Lueh, page 152. "A woman who feels as if a piece of broiled meat is stuck in her throat should take *Ban xia hou po tang* (Pinellia and Magnolia Combination)."

Ginseng and Gypsum Combination

Bai hu jia ren shen tang

Gypsum	*Gypsum Fibrosum*	*Shi gao*	15.0
Anemarrhena	*Anemarrhenae Rhizoma*	*Zhi mu*	5.0
Oryza	*Oryza Semen*	*Jing mi*	10.0
Licorice	*Glycyrrhizae Radix*	*Gan cao*	2.0
Ginseng	*Ginseng Radix*	*Ren shen*	3.0

This heat clearing formula is used for an average-strong person with either yin deficiency or excess yang causing both internal and external heat; symptoms include respiratory disorders, severe thirst, fever, severe chills and fatigue.

Functions:

Clears heat, cools the body, pacifies the spirit, relieves irritability, increases body fluids, and relieves thirst.

Main Conformations:

Extreme thirst, dry mouth and tongue, excessive sweating, chest discomfort and irritability, obstruction and hardness beneath the heart, abdomen soft yet full, hard stools, frequent urination, pain and heaviness in the extremities.

Major Indications:

1. Pulse; forceful, big or floating.
2. Tongue: red with thin or thick yellow coat; dry.
3. Abdomen: full, and soft.
4. Hot skin diseases.
5. Heatstroke.
6. Constipation.
7. Pneumonia.
8. Mental restlessness and irritability.
9. Kidney and gallbladder disorders.
10. Diabetes.

References from the Classics:

Shang Han Lun, page 8. "If severe perspiration, marked distress, prolonged thirst, and a large pulse persist after taking *Gui zhi tang* (Cinnamon Combination), *Bai hu jia ren shen tang* (Ginseng and Gypsum Combination) should be taken."

Shang Han Lun, pages 26-27. "*Bai hu jia ren shen tang* (Ginseng and Gypsum Combination) should be prescribed for patients with *shang han* conditions with a floating pulse, fever without perspiration, and thirst, but with no "surface" conformation. Those with surface conformations should never be treated with *Bai hu jia ren shen tang* (Ginseng and Gypsum Combination)."

Shang Han Lun, page 38. "Cases in which thirst and dryness of the mouth and tongue are present should be given *Bai hu jia ren shen tang* (Ginseng and Gypsum Combination)."

Chin Kuei Yao Lueh, page 18. "Heatstroke (*yeh*), a greater yang disease, manifests as sweating, chillphobia, generalized fever and thirst. *Bai hu jia ren shen tang* (Ginseng and Gypsum Combination) is the primary treatment."

Chin Kuei Yao Lueh, page 96. "A patient with thirst for water and a dry mouth and lips should drink *Bai hu jia ren shen tang* (Ginseng and Gypsum Combination)."

Lotus Seed Combination

Qing xin lian zi yin

Lotus Seed	*Nelumbonis Semen*	*Lian zi*	4.0
Ophiopogon	*Ophiopogonis Tuber*	*Mai men tong*	4.0
Hoelen	*Poria*	*Fu ling*	4.0
Ginseng	*Ginseng Radix*	*Ren shen*	3.0
Plantago	*Plantaginis Semen*	*Che qian zi*	3.0
Scute	*Scutellariae Radix*	*Huang qin*	3.0
Astragalus	*Astragali Radix*	*Huang qi*	2.0
Lycium Bark	*Lycii Radicis Cortex*	*Di gu pi*	2.0
Licorice	*Glycyrrhizae Radix*	*Gan cao*	2.0

This formula comes under the fire purging category, but it is important to remember that in this condition the heat is only in the upper jiao. The lower jiao is cold, so the formula is designed not only to purge heat in the upper jiao, but also harmonize the upper and lower jiaos; it nourishes the spleen, stomach and kidney, and dispels internal heat in the heart and lungs. Persons taking this formula are of delicate constitution, show heat rising, and have chronic disorders and general fatigue and weakness. *Qing xin lian zi yin* (Lotus Seed Combination) nourishes and regulates the yin, including the fluid aspect of the yin.

Functions:

Clears heart heat, dispels moisture, tonifies qi, nourishes yin, and supplements spleen and kidneys.

Main Conformations:

Excess symptoms in the upper part of the body, deficient symptoms in the lower part of the body, nervousness, extreme thirst, bitter taste in the mouth, dry throat, discomfort in the heart, and tired arms and legs.

Major Indications:

1. Pulse; weak, rapid, and thready or slippery.
2. Tongue; pale, flabby and dry or pasty (cotton mouth), possibly with a red dry patch in the center of the tongue, and possibly with sores on the tongue and elsewhere in mouth.
3. Abdomen: weak, sloshing, and flabby.
4. General fatigue.
5. Gastrointestinal weakness.
6. Chronic leukorrhea, and gonorrhea.
7. Diabetes mellitus.
8. Anorexia.
9. Dysuria, and cystitis.
10. Impotence.

Ophiopogon Combination

Mai men dong tang

Ophiopogon	*Ophiopogonis Tuber*	*Mai men tong*	10.0
Pinellia	*Pinellia Tuber*	*Ban xia*	5.0
Oryza	*Oryza Semen*	*Jing mi*	5.0
Jujube	*Zizyphi Fructus*	*Da zao*	3.0
Ginseng	*Ginseng Radix*	*Ren shen*	2.0
Licorice	*Glycyrrhizae Radix*	*Gan cao*	2.0

This moistening formula is mainly used in deficient lung yin conditions in an average-weak type person. The formula not only moistens, but cools the body; symptoms include flushingup, dry and irritated throat, dyspnea, spasmodic coughing, and hoarseness.

Functions:

Nourishes stomach fluid and subdues flushingup.

Main Conformations:

Dryness in the throat with sensation of pricking, spastic cough, scanty sputum, which is difficult to cough up, dry skin, and obstruction beneath the heart.

Major Indications:

1. Pulse; big, weak, and floating or sinking.
2. Tongue; red, no coat, or thick white or yellow coat.
3. Abdomen; obstruction beneath the heart, possibly hard or tense in the hypochondric region.
4. Asthma.
5. Dry, and bleeding throat.
6. Respiratory infections.
7. General yin deficient symptoms.

References from the Classics:

Chin Kuei Yao Lueh, page 52. "The patient with an adverse cough, flushingup of qi, and throat discomfort should be treated principally with *Mai men dong tang* (Ophiopogon Combination) in order to suppress the adversity and make qi descend."

Lily Combination

Bai he gu jin tang

Lily	*Lilii Bulbus*	*Bai he*	4.0
Peony	*Paeoniae Radix*	*Shao yao*	3.0
Tang-kuei	*Angelicae Radix*	*Dang gui*	4.0
Fritillaria	*Fritillariae Bulbus*	*Bei mu*	3.0
Licorice	*Glycyrrhizae Radix*	*Gan cao*	0.5
Rehmannia (cooked)	*Rehmanniae Radix*	*Shu di huang*	4.0
Ophiopogon	*Ophiopogonis Tuber*	*Mai men dong*	6.0
Scrophularia	*Scrophulariae Radix*	*Xuan shen*	3.0
Platycodon	*Platycodi Radix*	*Jie geng*	2.0

This formula acts as a tonic, antipyretic and expectorant, and nourishes the lungs and the kidneys. It removes internal heat from the lungs and dispels sputum.

Functions:

Nourishes yin, clears heat, strengthens lungs, and dispels phlegm.

Major Indications:

1. Pulse; thready and rapid.
2. Tongue; red tongue with little coating.
3. Abdomen: N/A.
4. Coughing and hemoptysis.
5. Pharyngitis.
6. Asthma and wheezing due to internal heat.
7. Hoarseness.

Ma-huang, Aconite and Asarum Combination

Ma huang xi xin fu zi tang

(AKA) Ma-huang and Asarum Combination

Ma huang fu zi xi xin tang

Aconite (processed)	*Aconiti Carmichaelii Praeparata Radix*	*Fu zi*	0.5-1.0
Asarum	*Asari Herba Cum Radice*	*Xi xin*	3.0
Ma-huang	*Ephedrae Herba*	*Ma huang*	4.0

This formula is used for treating overall exhaustion and achiness in very weak, debilitated, or old persons. The formula is warming and should only be used in a weak, cold, or deficient yang conformation. It is usually used in cases of acute onset of pathogenic wind/cold invasion.

Functions:

Restores yang, and dispels chill.

Main Conformations:

Anemic facial complexion, mild fever, lassitude, chills in the back and head, general aching, edema in legs, and cold arms and legs.

Major Indications:

1. Pulse; submerged and thready.
2. Tongue; pale, white coat.
3. Abdomen: water stagnancy.
4. Common cold in the elderly.
5. Wind/cold invasion causing upper respiratory disorders.
6. Headaches due to wind and cold.
7. Anemia and fatigue.
8. Edema.
9. Trigeminal neuralgia and headache.

References from the Classics:

Shang Han Lun, page 47. "For patients contracting lesser yin disease with fever (a symptom of lesser yang disease) and a sinking pulse, *Ma huang xi xin fu zi tang* (Ma-huang, Aconite and Asarum Combination) is indicated."

Vitality Combination

Zhen wu tang

Hoelen	*Poria*	*Fu ling*	5.0
Peony	*Paeoniae Radix*	*Shao yao*	3.0
Atractylodes (white)	*Atractylodis Rhizoma*	*Bai shu*	3.0
Ginger (fresh)	*Zingiberis Rhizoma*	*Sheng jiang*	3.0
Aconite (processed)	*Aconiti Carmichaelii Praeparata Radix*	*Fu zi*	0.5-1.0

This chill dispelling formula is used for deficiency disorders of metabolism or of the upper respiratory tract, which are associated most commonly with water stagnancy, generalized weakness, and fatigue.

Functions:

Supplements yang, warms the interior, promotes water metabolism and dispels stagnant water.

Main Conformations:

Weak yin conformation, tongue moist or with white or pale black fur, vomiting, chillphobia, cardiac herper function, abdomen soft and weak, clear or decreased urine, general lassitude and pain, cold hands and feet.

Major Indications:

1. Pulse; deep and minute, or floating and weak.
2. Tongue; moist, with white or pale black fur.
3. Abdomen; soft, weak, and distended; water palpable in the gastric region.
4. Respiratory disorders.
5. Gastrointestinal weakness.
6. General damp/cold symptoms; cold hands and feet.
7. Valvular diseases.
8. Edema due to nephritis.
9. Rheumatic pain.

References from the Classics:

Shang Han Lun, page 15-16. "If the patient continues to have a fever, rapid heart palpitation, vertigo, trembling, and a tendency to collapse after perspiring, which has been induced by the sweating method, he still has a greater yang disease and should be treated with *Zhen wu tang* (Vitality Combination), but the disease has entered the lesser yin conformation."

Shang Han Lun, page 50. "Lesser yin disease persisting for two-to-five days with abdominal discomfort, difficulty in urination, heaviness and aching of the limbs, diarrhea, cough, excessive urination, constipation, and vomiting should be treated with *Zhen wu tang* (Vitality Combination)."

Note: There are many versions of Shang Han Lun and Chin Kuei Yao Lueh in the Orient. Only a few translations exist in English. As referred to here, these two classics are the translations done by Dr. Hong-yen Hsu, Oriental Healing Arts Institute, Long Beach, California.

Shang Han Lun

Translation is taken from Shang Han Lun Cheih Shuo, 1966, written in Japanese by Otsuka Keisetsu in Kuo-ting. This was translated into English as Shang Han Lun The Great Classic of Chinese Medicine, translated and edited by Hong-yen Hsu, Ph.D., and William G. Peacher, M.D., Oriental Healing Arts Institute, Long Beach, California, 1981.

Chin Kuei Yao Lueh

This version of Chin Kuei yao Lueh is Chin Kuei Yao Lueh Chiang I published by the Wen Kuang Publishing Company, Taiwan. This was translated into English as Chin Kuei Yao Lueh a Chinese Medical Classic by Dr. Hong-yen Hsu and Su-yen Wang, Oriental Healing Arts Institute, Long Beach, California, 1983.

Chapter 4

DIGESTIVE DISORDERS

The following formulas are arranged in order from the stronger and more aggressive to the more nutritive. The order is not an absolute, but rather a basic guide to how the formulas can be arranged for treatment.

During the yang ming (second) stage of disease, when there are signs of internal heat toxins, the following formulas should be considered:

- Coptis & Rhubarb Combination
  (*Xie xin tang*)
- Major Rhubarb Combination
  (*Da cheng qi tang*)
- Persica & Rhubarb Combination
  (*Tao he cheng qi tang*)

During the shao yang (third) stage of disease, the following formulas should be considered:

- Pinellia and Magnolia Combination
  (*Ban xia hou po tang*)
- Pinellia Combination
  (*Ban xia xie xin tang*)
- Pinellia and Ginger Combination
  (*Sheng jiang xie xin tang*)

- Pinellia and Licorice Combination
  (*Gan cao xie xin tang*)
- Minor Pinellia and Hoelen Combination
  (*Xiao ban xia jia fu ling tang*)

During the tai yin (fourth) stage of disease, the following formulas should be considered:

- Four Major Herb Combination
  (*Si jun zi tang*)
- Six Major Herb Combination
  (*Liu jun zi tang*)
- Pinellia and Ginseng Six Combination
  (*Ban xie liu jun zi tang*)

During the jue yin (sixth) stage of disease, the following formulas should be considered:

- Ginseng and Astragalus Combination
  (*Bu zhong yi qi tang*)
- W.T.T.C.
  (*Le shi shu*)

Digestive Disorder Symptoms

The following are basic disorders and indications commonly treated with the formulas in this section.

Acute Gastritis

Symptoms: discomfort and stagnation in the stomach, vomiting, headache, severe chills, fever, and diarrhea.

Appendicitis

Symptoms: initially severe pain in the stomach which, after persisting thirty minutes to an hour, becomes localized in the lower right abdomen, and is accompanied by tenderness and rigidity over the right abdominis rectus muscle, or McBurney's point. When the patient stretches the right leg there is severe pain and tension which causes the abdominis rectus muscle to become rigid.

Ascites

Symptoms: subdermal veins of the abdomen become visible, cardiac palpitations increase, and breathing becomes labored as a result of the diaphragm being raised by the ascites.

Carcinoma of the Esophagus

Symptoms: progressive dysphagia, as the principal symptom, which ultimately prevents the swallowing of even liquids. Anterior or posterior chest pain which is unrelated to eating implies local extension of the tumor, and significant weight loss over a short period of time is an ominous sign.

Chronic Gastritis

Symptoms: either a feeling of heaviness in the stomach or chest distention, subcardiac pain after eating, impaired gastric function which can cause a decreased secretion of gastric juice, and abdominal muscle atrophy.

Esophageal Neurosis (Esophageal Spasm)

Symptoms: difficulty in swallowing, compressed sensation in the chest, labored breathing, cardiac palpitation, and an aching and burning sensation in the esophagus.

Esophageal Stenosis (Constriction of the Esophagus)

Symptoms: difficulty in swallowing which may not appear until years after an initial injury.

Esophagitis

Symptoms: burning sensation in the esophagus (pyrosis) which is often worsened by recumbency and ameliorated by antacids, and difficulty in swallowing; blood tinged regurgitated material or occasional vomiting of blood, anemia, and stricture formation are later manifestations.

Gastrectasis

Symptoms: indigestion, abdominal distention with succussion in the stomach, anorexia, nausea, vomiting, thirst, and a sensation of heavy pressure in the stomach.

Gastric Cancer

Symptoms: in general the initial stages of all cancers are asymptomatic. However, early warning signs may include weight loss, anorexia, a change of eating habits, stagnation in the stomach, nausea, abdominal pain, chest distention, and vomiting.

Gastroasthenia

Symptoms: anorexia, and a feeling of stagnation in the stomach. Other subjective symptoms are bloating, nausea, stomachache, stomach discomfort, vertigo, distress, emotional instability, irritability, impatience, tinnitus, insomnia, and nervousness.

Gastrointestinal Weakness

Symptoms: thin body, lack of vitality, tendency to be easily fatigued, diarrhea, slight abdominal pain, mild vertigo, palpitations, succussion in the abdomen, and sometimes rigid abdominal walls.

Gastroptosis

Symptoms: an abdomen which seems hollow between the ribs, and swelling in the lower abdomen. Other symptoms are heaviness in the head, insomnia, vertigo due to constipation, amnesia, anxiety, lack of vitality, and nervousness. When gastroptosis is accompanied by gastric disturbance, the patient will experience anorexia and stomachache.

Gastrospasm

Symptoms: a sudden severe pain in the upper abdomen which soon becomes spasmodic.

Gastroxnysis

Symptoms: feverish feeling in the stomach, chest distress, regurgitation of sour fluid, belching, and stomachache.

Laxity of the Stomach

Symptoms: sensation of gastric distention, obstruction of ingested foods in the stomach, belching, nausea, and a loss of appetite. Abdominal examination usually reveals splashing sounds.

Peptic Ulcer

Symptoms: severe stomachache, severe nausea, bloody sputum, dark tarry stools, stomach discomfort, sensation of stagnation in the stomach, and subcardiac pain.

Peritonitis

Symptoms: symptoms are divided into systemic reactions and abdominal signs.

Systemic reactions are: malaise, prostration, nausea, vomiting, septic fever, leukocytosis, and electrolyte imbalance.

Abdominal signs are: local or generalized pain, abdominal pain upon coughing, tenderness to light percussion over the inflamed peritonitis. Pelvic peritonitis is associated with rectal and vaginal tenderness.

Formulas for Digestive Disorders

Formula	Stage	Classification	Qi, Water blood	Disorder	Patient Type
Coptis and Rhubarb C.	shao yang/ yang ming	fire purging	qi	acute	strong
Major Rhubarb C.	yang ming	interior attacking	qi	acute	strong
Persica and Rhubarb C.	yang ming	blood	blood	chronic	strong
Pinellia and Magnolia C.	shao yang	qi	qi/ water	acute/ chronic	weak
Pinellia C.	shao yang/ tai yin	harmonizing	qi/ water	acute/ chronic	strong/ weak
Pinellia and Ginger C.	shao yang/ tai yin	harmonizing	water	acute	weak
Pinellia and Licorice C.	shao yang/ tai yin	harmonizing	qi/ water	chronic	weak
Minor Pinellia and Hoelen C.	tai yin	diuretic	water	acute	weak
Four Major Herb C.	tai yin	tonic	water	chronic	weak
Six Major Herb C.	tai yin	tonic	water	chronic	weak
Pinellia and Ginseng Six C.	tai yin	tonic	qi	chronic	weak
Ginseng and Astragalus C.	tai yin/ jue yin	tonic	qi	chronic	weak
W.T.T.C.	jue yin	carbuncle/ dermatosis	qi	chronic	weak

Coptis & Rhubarb Combination

Xie xin tang

Rhubarb	*Rhei Rhizoma*	*Da huang*	1.0
Scute	*Scutellariae Radix*	*Huang qin*	1.0
Coptis	*Coptidis Rhizoma*	*Huang lian*	1.0

This formula is more aggressive and cold than *Da cheng qi tang* (Major Rhubarb Combination), and is best used for patients in an acute stage of yang ming with a strong constitution. Symptoms include congestion of the digestive organs and flushingup.

Functions:

Clears heat, promotes evacuation, arrests bleeding, and pacifies the spirit.

Main Conformations:

Facial flushing, feeling of insecurity, tendency to be easily frightened, hemoptysis (fresh red bleeding from the nose), obstruction beneath the heart (soft on the surface and hard at the base), and constipation.

Major Indications:

1. Pulse; forceful.
2. Tongue; yellow coat.
3. Abdomen; distended, hard, and tense.
4. Constipation.
5. Stomach distention and congestion.
6. Flushingup.
7. Emotional instability, nervousness, and anxiety.

References from the Classics:

Chin Kuei Yao Lueh, page 120. "*Xie xin tang* (Coptis & Rhubarb Combination) treats patients with deficiency of heart qi, hematemesis, and nosebleeds."

Chin Kuei Yao Lueh, page 153. "A slobbering woman who undergoes purgation only and has, as a result, obstruction beneath the heart, should first be given *Xiao qing long tang* (Minor Blue Dragon Combination) to arrest the slobbering. After the slobbering has ceased, *Xie xin tang* (Coptis and Rhubarb Combination) will relieve the obstruction."

Major Rhubarb Combination

Da cheng qi tang

Rhubarb	*Rhei Rhizoma*	*Da huang*	2.0
Chih-shih	*Aurantii Fructus Immaturus*	*Zhi shi*	2.0
Mirabilitum	*Natrium Sulfuricum*	*Mang xiao*	2.0
Magnolia Bark	*Magnoliae Officinalis Cortex*	*Hou pu*	5.0

This formula is used to purge a strong person suffering from constipation, abdominal distention, moist fever, and a dry tongue and mouth. It is contraindicated in persons with a fast, weak, pulse and ascites.

Functions:

Purges accumulated interior heat, clears fire, and detoxifies.

Main Conformations:

Sunlight yang conformation, perspiration on face, arms and legs, delirium, chest discomfort and distress, extreme thirst with tidal fever, abdominal fullness, distention and pain upon palpation, and constipation.

Major Indications:

1. Pulse; deep and strong, or quick and slippery.
2. Tongue; red and dry with black or brown fur, usually red dots at the back of the tongue.
3. Abdomen; full, distended, and firm with pain or palpitation.
4. Hypertension.
5. Obesity.
6. Habitual constipation, especially with abdominal fullness.
7. Heaviness in the body.
8. Pneumonia.
9. Mental delirium.

References from the Classics:

Shang Han Lun, page 35. "Sunlight yang disease with a slow but strong pulse, perspiration but no severe chills, heaviness of the body which makes motion difficult, rapid respiration, stomach congestion, stridor due to pressure in the chest, tidal fever, and perspiration of the hands and feet should be treated primarily with *Da cheng qi tang* (Major Rhubarb Combination)."

Shang Han Lun, page 36. "In severe cases of *shang han* condition the patient may fail to recognize others, be easily frightened, have purposeless movements, restlessness, slight gasping respiration, fixed staring, and delirium. This indicates the need for *Da cheng qi tang* (Major Rhubarb Combination)."

Shang Han Lun, page 36. "Sunlight yang disease accompanied by delirium and tidal fever suggests a *Da cheng qi tang* (Major Rhubarb Combination) conformation."

Shang Han Lun, page 57. "The complications of greater and sunlight yang disease, when the greater yang surface conformation has been relieved but the sunlight inside conformation continues, exhibits symptoms of tidal fever, severe perspiration on the hands and feet, constipation, and delirium, which will be relieved by the purgation method and *Da cheng qi tang* (Major Rhubarb Combination)."

Shang Han Lun, page 40. "If...there are...dry stools due to heat and firmness, *Da cheng qi tang* (Major Rhubarb Combination) should be given."

Shang Han Lun, page 41. "*Shang han* conditions that prevail for six to seven days...causing blurred vision, disturbed ocular function, absence of surface and interior conformation,and mild body fever, should be purged without delay with *Da cheng qi tang* (Major Rhubarb Combination)."

"A combination of sunlight and lesser yang diseases with diarrhea, smooth and rapid pulse, and undigested food remaining in the stomach can be purged with an alternate treatment of *Da cheng qi tang* (Major Rhubarb Combination)."

Shang Han Lun, page 51. "Immediate purging with *Da cheng qi tang*

(Major Rhubarb Combination) is recommended for lesser yin disease with watery, clear, greenish colored diarrhea, aching beneath the heart with palpitations, and dryness of the mouth."

Chin Kuei Yao Lueh, page 13. "A strong convulsive disease in a patient manifesting thoracic fullness, lockjaw, tetany, spasm of the feet, and involuntary gnashing of teeth may be treated with *Da cheng qi tang* (Major Rhubarb Combination)."

Chin Kuei Yao Lueh, page 68. "Abdominal distention which remains unreduced, or only slightly reduced, should be purged with *Da cheng qi tang* (Major Rhubarb Combination) as the preferred drug."

Chin Kuei Yao Lueh, page 72. "A quick and slippery pulse reflects fullness from the presence of overnight undigested food. It can be purged principally with *Da cheng qi tang* (Major Rhubarb Combination)."

Chin Kuei Yao Lueh, page 129. "Diarrhea with a slow and slippery pulse signifies a firm condition of the stomach. If the diarrhea shows no sign of ceasing, the person should be purged immediately with *Da cheng qi tang* (Major Rhubarb Combination) as the preferred formula."

Chin Kuei Yao Lueh, page 130. "In diarrhea, a slippery pulse signifies that purging will cure the patient. The remedy called for is *Da cheng qi tang* (Major Rhubarb Combination)."

Chin Kuei Yao Lueh, page 146. "If a woman regains her appetite after taking *Xiao chai hu tang* (Minor Bupleurum Combination), but has a relapse of fever seven or eight days later, she has gastric firmness and primarily needs *Da cheng qi tang* (Major Rhubarb Combination)."

Chin Kuei Yao Lueh, page 147. "If a woman develops hardening and aching in the lower abdomen, but no greater yang symptoms seven or eight days after labor, she has not completely discharged the lochia. However, a minute and full pulse, constipation, discomfort and irritation with fever and no appetite--the discomfort, irritation, and fever becoming more severe toward dusk--and delirium occurring after eating but disappearing at night signals that a fever has stagnated in the interior and is bound to the urinary bladder. Such a woman requires *Da cheng qi tang* (Major Rhubarb Combination)."

Persica & Rhubarb Combination

Tao he cheng qi tang

Persica	*Persicae Semen*	*Tao ren*	5.0
Rhubarb	*Rhei Rhizoma*	*Da huang*	3.0
Cinnamon Twigs	*Cinnamomi Ramulus*	*Gui zhi*	4.0
Mirabilitum	*Natrium Sulfuricum*	*Mang xiao*	2.0
Licorice	*Glycyrrhizae Radix*	*Gan cao*	1.5

This formula is primarily used for treating stagnant blood in the lower jiao in persons of strong constitution. Generally speaking the disease will be long standing since it is on a blood level, and one will often see marked flushingup.

Functions:

Disperses stagnant blood and lumps in the abdomen.

Main Conformations:

Occluded blood, strong conformation, over excitability, hysteria, tinnitus with vertigo, dry mouth, flushingup with redness around the nose, general burning sensation, pulsation of the abdominal artery, sensation of distention in the lower abdomen, pain in the lower abdomen and lower back, constipation, spasms with cold legs and feet, and uterine bleeding.

Major Indications:

1. Pulse; deep and tight, or floating.
2. Tongue; red or purple with yellow coat.
3. Abdomen; distended with cramping and pain in the lower jiao, pain on palpation, and pulsation of the abdominal artery.
4. Constipation.
5. Urogenital disorders due to stagnant blood.
6. Bleeding.
7. Hypertension.
8. Emotional instability.
9. Skin diseases due to heat in the blood.

10. Headache, vertigo, and tinnitus.
11. Low back pain.
12. Spasms, and cold hands and feet.

References from the Classics:

Shang Han Lun, page 18. "An unrelieved greater yang disease that exhibits a feverish lower jiao (the area between the stomach and the bladder) will result in extravasated blood, which, in turn, will cause delirium in the patient. This condition may be helped by eliminating the extravasated blood from a bloody stool. However, if the surface symptoms do not improve, with or without a bloody stool, purgative herbs should not be further administered. The surface symptoms should be relieved first, and when this is done the acute lower abdominal pain may be dispersed with *Dao he cheng qi tang* (Persica and Rhubarb Combination)."

Pinellia and Magnolia Combination

Ban xia hou po tang

Pinellia	*Pinellia Tuber*	*Ban xia*	6.0
Magnolia Bark	*Magnoliae Officinalis Cortex*	*Hou pu*	3.0
Hoelen	*Poria*	*Fu ling*	5.0
Ginger (fresh)	*Zingiberis Rhizoma*	*Sheng jiang*	4.0
Perilla Leaves	*Perillae Folium*	*Zi su ye*	2.0

This formula is used for stagnation in the stomach and chest, weak gastrointestinal tract, and a weak overall constitution.

Functions:

Regulates qi, disperses stagnancy, subdues flushingup, and dispels stagnant phlegm and water.

Main Conformations:

Weak gastrointestinal tract, water stagnation in the stomach, sensation of something stuck in the throat (globus hystericus), facial edema with anemia, vomiting, cough with asthma, chest pain, depression with restlessness, glassy eyes, fatigue, and decreased urine.

Major Indications:

1. Pulse; floating and weak, or sunken and thin.
2. Tongue; pale.
3. Abdomen; weak with water sloshing sounds.
4. Gastrointestinal weakness with abdominal fullness.
5. Emotional instability and stress reactions.
6. Muscle and skin flaccidity.
7. Flushingup.

References from the Classics:

Chin Kuei Yao Lueh, page 152. "A woman who feels as if a piece of broiled meat is stuck in her throat should take *Ban xia hou po tang* (Pinellia & Magnolia Combination)."

Pinellia Combination

Ban xia xie xin tang

Pinellia	*Pinellia Tuber*	*Ban xia*	6.0
Scute	*Scutellariae Radix*	*Huang qin*	3.0
Coptis	*Coptidis Rhizoma*	*Huang lian*	1.0
Ginseng	*Ginseng Radix*	*Ren shen*	3.0
Jujube	*Zizyphi Fructus*	*Da zao*	3.0
Ginger (dried)	*Zingiberis Siccatum Rhizoma*	*Gan jiang*	3.0
Licorice	*Glycyrrhizae radix*	*Gan cao*	3.0

This is a harmonizing formula which is used for treating gastrointestinal disease in weak or strong persons. Symptoms include expansion and/or inflammation in the gastrointestinal tract, and a perception of fullness in the hypochondriac area.

Functions:

Clears stomach and intestines of dampness and heat, and strengthens the functions of the stomach and intestines.

Main Conformations:

Nausea, vomiting, restlessness, loss of appetite, water stagnation in the stomach, borborygmus, and diarrhea.

Major Indications:

1. Pulse; flooding, and slippery.
2. Tongue; white coat, flabby, and swollen.
3. Abdomen; perceivable water stagnancy in the stomach.
4. Gastrointestinal disorders.
5. Nausea and vomiting.
6. Loss of appetite.
7. Ulcers.
8. Motion sickness.

References from the Classics:

Shang Han Lun, page 23. "For cases of congestion beneath the heart without pain, *Ban xia xie xin tang* (Pinellia Combination) is recommended."

Shang Han Lun, page 25. "If incessant diarrhea, stagnancy, and hardness beneath the heart have resulted following treatment with some purgatory herb for the *shang han* condition, further treatment with pinellia formulas, such as *Gan cao xia xin tang* (Pinellia and Licorice Combination), Sheng jian xie xin tang (Pinellia and Ginger Combination), or *Ban xia xie xin tang* (Pinellia Combination) followed by other purgatives fails to stop incessant diarrhea, or is further aggravated by the physician's treatment with *Ren shen tang* (Ginseng and Ginger Combination), the patient should then be mainly given *Chi shi zhi yu yu liang tang* (Kaolin and Limonite Combination)."

Chin Kuei Yao Lueh page 123. "*Ban xia xie xin tang* (Pinellia Combination) treats vomiting accompanied by borborygmus and obstruction beneath the heart."

Sheng jiang xie xin tang (Pinellia and Ginger Combination) is the same as *Ban xia xie xin tang* (Pinellia Combination) except the amount of dried ginger is decreased and the amount of raw ginger is increased, making the formula warmer and more aggressive. This formula is used to treat weak stomach qi, stagnant food in the stomach, and moisture in the chest and abdomen; the most common symptoms are vomiting, nausea, and dampness and stagnancy especially in the middle jiao.

Pinellia and Ginger Combination

Sheng jiang xie xin tang

Pinellia	*Pinellia Tuber*	*Ban xia*	5.0
Scute	*Scutellariae Radix*	*Huang qin*	2.5
Licorice	*Glycyrrhizae Radix*	*Gan cao*	2.5
Ginseng	*Ginseng Radix*	*Ren shen*	2.5
Jujube	*Zizyphi Fructus*	*Da zao*	2.5
Coptis	*Coptidis Rhizoma*	*Huang lian*	1.0
Ginger (dried)	*Zingiberis Siccatum Rhizoma*	*Gan jiang*	1.5
Ginger (fresh)	*Zingiberis Rhizoma*	*Sheng-jiang*	2.0

Functions:

Clears moisture and heat from the stomach and intestines, strengthens the functions of the stomach and intestines, relieves qi stagnancy, and promotes digestion.

Main Conformations:

Nausea, vomiting, stagnation of water in the stomach, gastric discomfort, obstruction and hardening beneath the heart, acid regurgitation, borborygmus, and diarrhea.

Major Indications:

1. Pulse; flooding and rolling, or possibly large and floating at the bar positions.
2. Tongue; thickly coated, swollen, and/or moist body.
3. Abdomen; water stagnancy beneath the heart and in the stomach region.
4. Gastrointestinal disorders.
5. Diarrhea.
6. Vomiting.
7. Obstruction beneath the heart.

References from the Classics:

Shang Han Lun, page 24. "If there is impairment of digestion, hardness beneath the heart, retching, fluid below the ribs, and borborygmus with diarrhea, *Sheng jiang xie xin tang* (Pinellia and Ginger Combination) should be administered."

***Chin Kuei Yao Lueh*,** page 126. "*Sheng jiang xie xin tang* (Pinellia & Ginger Combination) relieves dry heaves, regurgitation, and frothy salivation."

Pinellia and Licorice Combination

Gan cao xie xin tang

Pinellia	*Pinellia Tuber*	*Ban xia*	5.0
Scute	*Scutellariae Radix*	*Huang qin*	2.5
Ginger (dried)	*Zingiberis Siccatum Rhizoma*	*Gan jiang*	2.5
Ginseng	*Ginseng Radix*	*Ren shen*	2.5
Jujube	*Zizyphi Fructus*	*Da zao*	2.5
Licorice	*Glycyrrhizae Radix*	*Gan cao*	2.5
Coptis	*Coptidis Rhizoma*	*Huang lian*	1.0

This formula is used for stress related gastrointestinal complaints with symptoms of distention beneath the heart, borborygmus, diarrhea, nausea, and mental stress and instability.

Functions:

Harmonizes stomach, subdues ascending qi, clears the heart, and pacifies the mind.

Main Conformations:

Mental instability (impetuousness), loss of appetite, gasping, obstruction beneath the heart with annoyance above, and diarrhea more than ten times a day.

Major Indications:

1. Pulse; rolling.
2. Tongue; swollen and white coat.
3. Abdomen; hardening at the hypochondric region.
4. Gastrointestinal disorders, especially when exacerbated by stress.
5. Nervous exhaustion and insomnia.
6. Stomatitis.

References from the Classics:

Chin Kuei Yao Lueh, page 24. "*Hu huo* disease resembles *shang han* disease in that the patient looks moribund, is somnolent and unable to close his eyes, and is so restless that he continually lies down and gets up. An ulcer in the larynx is *huo* disease, while an ulcer on the pudentum or the anus is *hu* disease. The patient, who is repelled by the odor of food, will be anorexic, and his facial color will vary from red to dark or pale. If ulcers develop in the upper part of the body, hoarseness occurs. The condition should principally be treated with *Gan cao xie xin tang* (Pinellia and Licorice Combination)."

Minor Pinellia and Hoelen Combination

Xiao ban xia jia fu ling tang

Pinellia	*Pinellia Tuber*	*Ban xia*	8.0
Ginger (fresh)	*Zingiberis Rhizoma*	*Sheng jiang*	5.0
Hoelen	*Poria*	*Fu ling*	5.0

This is a warming formula which is used to treat water stagnancy and toxins in the middle jiao in strong or weak persons.

Functions:

Dispels moisture and phlegm, harmonizes the stomach, and subdues flushingup.

Main Conformations:

Head sweating, vertigo, vomiting, extreme thirst, cardiac hyperfunction, obstruction and fullness beneath the heart, water stagnation in the stomach, decreased urine, and mild chills in the hands and feet.

Major Indications:

1. Pulse; thin.
2. Tongue; pale.
3. Abdomen: stagnant water in the stomach.
4. Pernicious vomiting.
5. Acute gastroenteritis.
6. Gastroptosis.

7. Vertigo.

8. Extreme thirst and decreased urination.

References from the Classics:

Chin Kuei Yao Lueh pages 87, 92. "The conformation of sudden vomiting, distention beneath the heart, water at the diaphragm, dizziness, and palpitation, should be treated essentially with *Xiao ban xia jia fu ling tang* (Minor Pinellia and Hoelen Combination)."

"A patient who initially manifests thirst followed by vomiting has stagnant water beneath the heart, and should be treated primarily with *Xiao ban xia jia fu ling tang* (Minor Pinellia and Hoelen Combination)."

Four Major Herb Combination

Si jun zi tang

Ginseng	*Ginseng Radix*	*Ren shen*	4.0
Atractylodes (white)	*Atractylodis Rhizoma*	*Bai shu*	4.0
Hoelen	*Poria*	*Fu ling*	4.0
Licorice	*Glycyrrhizae Radix*	*Gan cao*	1.5

This formula is used to treat gastrointestinal weakness in weak persons with loss of appetite, borborygmus, pallid complexion, weak abdomen, and weakness of the arms and legs. *Si jun zi tang* (Four Major Herb Combination) tonifies the qi of the spleen and stomach.

Functions:

Tonifies qi, and strengthens spleen.

Main Conformations:

Weak conformation, facial pallor, loss of voice, vomiting, weak gastrointestinal tract with water stagnation, abdominal weakness, borborygmus, diarrhea, and lassitude in the arms and legs.

Major Indications:

1. Pulse; weak, minute, or empty.
2. Tongue; pale and flabby.
3. Abdomen; weak, flaccid, and water sounds in the stomach.
4. Fatigue and anemia.

5. Gastrointestinal weakness and disorders.
6. Muscle weakness.
7. Diarrhea.
8. Bleeding.
9. Vomiting.
10. Enuresis.

Six Major Herb Combination

Liu jun zi tang

Ginseng	*Ginseng Radix*	*Ren shen*	4.0
Atractylodes (white)	*Atractylodis Rhizoma*	*Bai shu*	4.0
Hoelen	*Poria*	*Fu ling*	4.0
Pinellia	*Pinellia Tuber*	*Ban xia*	4.0
Citrus	*Citri Leiocarpae Exocarpium*	*Chen pi*	2.0
Ginger (fresh)	*Zingiberis Rhizoma*	*Sheng jiang*	2.0
Jujube	*Zizyphi Fructus*	*Da zao*	2.0
Licorice	*Glycyrrhizae Radix*	*Gan cao*	1.0

This formula is similar to *Si jun zi tang* (Four Major Herb Combination) in that it treats gastrointestinal weakness on a tai yin level with a symptom of stomach water stagnation. The difference is that while Four Major Herb Combination is aggressive and for persons with a stronger constitution (and perhaps more acute conditions), *Liu jun zi tang* (Six Major Herb Combination) is for older, colder, and weaker patients with more chronic conditions.

Functions:

Tonifies qi, strengthens spleen, dispels moisture,and prevents vomiting.

Main Conformations:

Weak conformation, anemia, loss of appetite, fatigue, pain in the shoulders, obstruction beneath the heart, weak gastrointestinal tract with water stagnation, abdominal laxity, and cold arms and legs.

Major Indications:

1. Pulse; weak.
2. Tongue; pale and flabby; in extreme cases, coated brown or black.
3. Abdomen; weak with water sounds in the stomach.
4. Chronic gastrointestinal disorders (including ulcers and cancer).
5. Fatigue and nervous exhaustion.
6. Cold limbs.
7. Distention beneath the heart.
8. Toxemia in pregnancy.

Pinellia and Ginseng Six Combination

Ban xie liu jun zi tang

Ginseng	*Ginseng Radix*	*Ren shen*	3.0
Atractylodes (white)	*Atractylodis Rhizoma*	*Bai shu*	3.0
Hoelen	*Poria*	*Fu ling*	3.0
Licorice	*Glycyrrhizae Radix*	*Gan cao*	3.0
Pinellia	*Pinellia Tuber*	*Ban xia*	3.0
Citrus	*Citri Leiocarpae Exocarpium*	*Chen pi*	3.0
Ginger (dried)	*Zingiberis Siccatum Rhizoma*	*Gan jiang*	3.0
Scute	*Scutellariae Radix*	*Huang qin*	3.0
Coptis	*Coptidis Rhizoma*	*Huang lian*	3.0
Oyster Shell	*Ostreae Testa*	*Mu li*	3.0

Ban xie liu jun zi tang (Pinellia and Ginseng Six Combination) is a tonifying formula that can be used in a broad fashion. It is effective in treating chronic gastrointestinal disorders in weak persons when caused by insufficient sleep, imbalanced diet, and overwork (i.e., depletion of qi).

Functions:

Strengthens spleen, dispels dampness, clears heat, and harmonizes stomach.

Main Conformation:

Weak conformation, weak gastrointestinal tract, cold arms and legs, loss of appetite, fatigue, obstruction beneath the heart, water stagnancy in the stomach, borborygmus, anemia, pain in the shoulders, weak pulse, restlessness, nausea and vomiting, diarrhea, and tongue coated with white fur.

Major Indications:

1. Pulse; weak, slow, deep, or empty.
2. Tongue; pale, swollen, and with thick white or yellow coat; or alternately, red.
3. Abdomen; weak, full, and soft.
4. Acute and chronic gastrointestinal disorders.
5. Abdominal distention, and dyspepsia.
6. Diarrhea.
7. Organ prolapse.

Ginseng and Astragalus Combination

Bu zhong yi qi tang

Astragalus	*Astragali Radix*	*Huang qi*	4.0
Ginseng	*Ginseng Radix*	*Ren shen*	4.0
Licorice	*Glycyrrhizae Radix*	*Gan cao*	1.5
Atractylodes (white)	*Atractylodis Rhizoma*	*Bai shu*	4.0
Citrus	*Citri Leiocarpae Exocarpium*	*Chen pi*	2.0
Tang-kuei	*Angelicae Radix*	*Dang gui*	3.0
Cimicifuga	*Cimicifugae Rhizoma*	*Sheng ma*	1.0
Bupleurum	*Bupleuri Radix*	*Chai hu*	2.0
Ginger (fresh)	*Zingiberis Rhizoma*	*Sheng jiang*	2.0
Jujube	*Zizyphi Fructus*	*Da zao*	2.0

This is a nourishing formula which is used to treat very weak persons with qi and water imbalance affecting the shao yin and tai yin levels of the body. The patient will display signs of both yin and yang deficiency, such as decreased gastrointestinal function, general fatigue, night sweats, and anorexia.

Functions:

Tonifies qi and strengthens the function of stomach and spleen.

Main Conformations:

Weak conformation, lifeless expression in the eyes, mild fever, loss of voice, loss of appetite, white froth in the mouth, desire for hot foods, spontaneous sweats, night sweats, abdominal laxity with palpitations beside the umbilicus, and tired arms and legs.

Major Indications:

1. Pulse; thin, soft, and weak.
2. Tongue; pale, or red, depending on dominant symptom picture; possible thin white coat, or peeling fur.
3. Abdomen; weak and with palpitation at the navel.
4. Extreme fatigue.
5. Organ prolapse.
6. Night sweats, spontaneous sweating.
7. Loss of appetite and weight.
8. Weak gastrointestinal tract.
9. Obesity due to excess water.
10. Chronic "damp" disorders.

W.T.T.C.

Le shi shu

Coix	*Coicis Semen*	*Yi yi ren*	10
Wisteria	*Wisteria Galla*	*Fugikofu*	10
Trapa	*Trapae Fructus*	*Ling jiao*	10
Terminalia	*Chebulae Fructus*	*Ke zi*	10

Le shi shu (W.T.T.C.) is specifically used for gastric and rectal cancer. It has a 40% cure rate according to a study done by Professor Nagayama of Chiba University in China. This formula inhibits the growth of cancer cells and prevents metastases after cancer surgery.

Functions:

Reduces inflammation, relieves pain, and inhibits cancer and rectal cancer (according to reports of a Ciba University study).

Major Indications:

1. Pulse: fast, wiry.
2. Tongue: possibly red.
3. Abdomen: deep aching pain.
4. Cancer of the intestines, rectum, and stomach.
5. Inflammation.
6. Dysuria and edema.
7. Arthralgia.
8. Suppuration (pus formation and discharge).
9. Pain and muscle spasm.

Chapter 5

KIDNEY AND UROLOGICAL DISORDERS

The following formulas are arranged in order from the stronger and more aggressive to the more nutritive. The order is not meant as an absolute, but rather as a basic guide to how the formulas can be arranged for treatment.

During the yang ming (third) stage of disease, where there is damp heat in the bladder, the following formulas could be considered:

- Gentiana Combination
  (*Long dan xie gan tang*)

- Polyporus Combination
  (*Zhu ling tang*)

When there is disharmony between the liver and kidneys, which causes water imbalance during the shao yang/shao yin stages, the following formulas should be considered:

- Bupleurum and Peony Formula
  (*Jia wei xiao yao san*)

- Bupleurum and Hoelen Combination
  (*Chai ling tang*)

- Hoelen Five Herb Formula
  (*Wu ling san*)
- Tang-kuei and Peony Formula
  (*Dang gui shao yao san*)

Kidney and Urological Disorder Symptoms

Listed below are the basic disorders and indications commonly treated with the formulas in this section.

Acute Nephritis

Symptoms: sore throat and fever. After ten to twenty days the above symptoms will disappear, but the patient remains tired, has low back pain, tendency towards fatigue, thirst, loss of appetite, albuminuria, hematuria, and sometimes edema.

Chronic Nephritis

Symptoms: in the primary stage there may be no symptoms of which the patient is aware. When the patient is ill or weak, edema will be present, but some patients will have albuminuria without edema. As the disease progresses, there will be an increase in blood pressure, pallor, blurred vision, palpitations, gasping respiration, and nocturia. In severe cases uremia and death will follow.

Degenerative Nephritis

Symptoms: loss of appetite, albuminuria, decrease in urinary output, and more marked edema than that in chronic nephritis.

Kidney Stones (Renal Calculi)

Symptoms: severe pain due to increased inner pressure in the renal pelvis, hematuria, occasional vomiting, and swollen abdomen. Paroxymal pain at the lower abdomen is called nephrocolic. Nephrocolic pain lasts about thirty minutes and then subsides.

Orchitis (Epididymitis)

Symptoms: swelling of the testes and scrotum, intense pain, chills with persistent high fever, hiccups, and vomiting.

Pyelitis

Symptoms: sudden onset with severe chills and shivering, fever, dull pain on both sides of the abdomen, frequent and increased urination, turbid urine, and albuminuria.

Renal Atrophy

Symptoms: pain, strangury, turbid urine, sensation of residual urine, and frequent urge to void. In severe cases there may be fever with the urine becoming reddish in color.

Urethral Calculi

Symptoms: renal calculi and urethral calculi bring about drastic paroxysmal abdominal pain starting from the sides of the kidneys and radiating, in turn, toward the bladder, urethra, and thighs. This progression is accompanied by nausea and vomiting.

Vesicle calculi cause pain upon urination, increases the frequency of urination, or, at times, a complete stoppage of urination. Urine is turbid, and symptoms are aggravated by physical exercise.

Urethritis

Symptoms: in the male there is urethral prurital itching, burning sensation on urination, lack of control of urination, and dysuria. In the female there is reddening of the external urethra, discharge of pus, burning sensation during urination, mild pain, and frequent urination.

Formulas for Kidney and Urological Disorders

Formula	Stage	Classification	Water Blood	Disorder	Patient Type
Gentiana C.	yang ming	fire purging	blood	acute	strong
Polyporus C.	yang ming	diuretic	water	acute	strong
Bupleurum and Peony C.	shao yang	harmonizing	blood	acute	strong
Bupleurum and Hoelen C.	shao yang/ shao yin	diuretic	water	chronic	weak
Hoelen Five C.	shao yang/ shao yin	diuretic	water	acute	weak
Tang-kuei and Peony C.	yang ming/ shao yin	gynecological	blood	chronic	weak

Gentiana Combination

Long dan xie gan tang

Gentiana	*Gentianae Scabrae Radix*	*Long dan*	1.0
Alisma	*Alismatis Rhizoma*	*Ze xie*	3.0
Akebia	*Akebiae Caulis*	*Mu tong*	5.0
Plantago	*Plantaginis Semen*	*Che qian zi*	3.0
Tang-kuei	*Angelicae Radix*	*Dang gui*	5.0
Rehmannia (raw)	*Rehmanniae Radix*	*Sheng di huang*	5.0
Gardenia	*Gardeniae Fructus*	*Zhi zi*	1.0
Scute	*Scutellariae Radix*	*Huang qie*	3.0
Licorice	*Glycyrrhizae Radix*	*Gan cao*	1.0

This is a fire purging formula which is used for persons with a strong to average constitution; it is contraindicated for persons with a delicate constitution. Its action is to eliminate heat and inflammation, and should be administered only briefly. It is best for acute flare-ups of true heat signs with symptoms of liver yang rising, heat in the blood, or dampness/heat in the lower jiao. Symptoms also include pain in the armpits, deafness, swollen ears, blood in the urine, and redness of the mouth and eyes.

Functions:

Clears liver heat and dampness.

Main Conformations:

Strong conformation, pale dark skin, tension and hypersensitivity on the outside of the abdominal rectus muscle, pain and swelling in the lower abdomen, and dampness on the inside of the hands and feet.

Major Indications:

1. Pulse; tense, rapid, forceful, and rolling.
2. Tongue; red with thick yellow coat.
3. Abdomen; tension, pain, and swelling in the lower abdomen.
4. Acute leukorrhea.
5. Gonorrhea, endometritis.

6. Hematuria, cystitis, and urethritis.
7. Herpes.
8. Itching, inflammation, and pain in the genital area.
9. Eczema, orchitis.

Polyporus Combination

Zhu ling tang

Polyporus	*Polyporus*	*Zhu ling*	3.0
Hoelen	*Poria*	*Fu ling*	3.0
Alisma	*Alismatis Rhizoma*	*Ze xie*	3.0
Talc	*Talcum and Kaolinum*	*Hua shi*	3.0
Gelatin	*Asini Gelatinum*	*A jiao*	3.0

This formula has diuretic action and is used to treat urinary difficulties, lower abdominal tension and fever, thirst, fever, vomiting, anxiety, and insomnia. It moistens dryness and dispels fever.

Functions:

Nourishes yin and dispels water stagnancy.

Main Conformations:

Insomnia, neurosis, fever, extreme thirst, flushingup of qi with chest discomfort, tension in the lower abdomen (toxic heat in the lower *jiao*), diarrhea, edema in the legs, decreased urine, and painful urination.

Major Indications:

1. Pulse; floating and rapid.
2. Tongue; red/dry and possibly with dark yellow fur–especially at the rear of the tongue.
3. Abdomen; tension, with fullness and pain in lower abdomen.
4. Nephritis, urethritis, and cystitis.
5. Gonorrhea.
6. External or internal bleeding.
7. Edema.
8. Diarrhea.

References from the Classics:

Shang Han Lun, page 50. "Patients with lesser yin disease characterized by persistent diarrhea lasting six or seven days, coughing, vomiting, thirst, anxiety, and insomnia, should be treated with *Zhu ling tang* (Polyporus Combination) (in order to moisten dryness and dispel fever)."

Shang Han Lun, page 38. "*Zhu ling tang* (Polyporus Combination) is recommended for patients with thirst and dysuria."

Chin Kuei Yao Lueh, page 9. "To treat visceral disease, prescribe a formula in accordance with the whole condition. For instance, if a person is thirsty, the formula *Zhu ling tang* (Polyporus Combination) will quench the thirst. This rule applies to all conditions."

Chin Kuei Yao Lueh, page 96. "A patient with a floating pulse, fever, thirst for water, and oliguria should be treated essentially with *Zhu ling tang* (Polyporus Combination)."

Bupleurum and Peony Formula

Jia wei xiao yao san

Tang-kuei	*Angelicae Radix*	*Dang gui*	3.0
Peony	*Paeoniae Radix*	*Shao yao*	3.0
Gardenia	*Gardeniae Fructus*	*Zhi zi*	2.0
Atractylodes (white)	*Atractylodis Rhizoma*	*Bai shu*	3.0
Hoelen	*Poria*	*Fu ling*	3.0
Mentha	*Menthae Herba*	*Bo he*	1.0
Bupleurum	*Bupleuri Radix*	*Chai hu*	3.0
Moutan	*Moutan Radicis Cortex*	*Mu dan pi*	2.0
Ginger (dried)	*Zingiberis Siccatum Rhizoma*	*Gan jiang*	1.0
Licorice	*Glycyrrhizae Radix*	*Gan cao*	2.0

This is a harmonizing formula which has a broad spectrum of uses including gynecological disorders, aching of the arms and legs, mental instability, flushingup, dizziness, insomnia, thirst, and abdominal distention; all of which are due to stagnant blood. The *Japanese Medical News* at one time reported that this formula was the best remedy for cirrhosis, abdominal tenseness, thirst with persistent and bitter taste in mouth, headache, turbid urine, and nosebleed.

Functions:

Soothes liver, removes liver qi stagnancy, tonifies spleen and blood, purges excess fire, and regulates menstruation.

Main Conformations:

Mild thoracocostal distress, afternoon flushingup sensation, vertigo, facial flushing, irritability, insomnia, feverish feeling that seems to move around, abnormal menstruation, and lassitude of the arms and legs,

Major Indications:

1. Pulse; tight, tense.
2. Tongue; purple or red dots.
3. Abdomen; tight.
4. Premenstrual syndrome (PMS).
5. Irregular menses, and infertility.
6. Menopausal symptoms.
7. Leukorrhea.
8. Constipation.
9. Acute and chronic damp heat infections in the urogenital tract (e.g., urethritis and cystitis).

Bupleurum and Hoelen Combination

Chai ling tang

Bupleurum	*Bupleuri Radix*	*Chai hu*	5.0
Pinellia	*Pinellia Tuber*	*Ban xia*	4.0
Scute	*Scutellariae Radix*	*Huang qin*	2.5
Ginseng	*Ginseng Radix*	*Ren shen*	2.5
Jujube	*Zizyphi Fructus*	*Da Zao*	2.5
Ginger (fresh)	*Zingiberis Rhizoma*	*Sheng jiang*	4.0
Licorice	*Glycyrrhizae Radix*	*Gan cao*	2.0
Cinnamon Twigs	*Cinnamomi Ramulus*	*Gui zhi*	2.5
Polyporus	*Polyporus*	*Zhu ling*	2.5
Atractylodes (white)	*Atractylodis Rhizoma*	*Bai shu*	2.5
Hoelen	*Poria*	*Fu ling*	2.5
Alisma	*Alismatis Rhizoma*	*Ze xie*	4.0

Chai ling tang (Bupleurum and Hoelen Combination) is a mixture of *Xiao chai hu tang* (Minor Bupleurum Combination) and *Wu ling san* (Hoelen Five Herb Formula). It is a harmonizing formula which is used to treat the symptoms of the above mentioned formulas as well as thirst, edema, dysuria, and diarrhea. The conformation of the patient will be of water and/or blood disharmony, and mainly affecting the liver and kidney energies. This formula is safe enough to take over a long period of time.

Functions:

Dispels stagnant water, strengthens spleen, and harmonizes lesser yang disease.

Major Indications:

1. Pulse; tight and full or wiry, or possibly floating.
2. Tongue; thick white coat, and it may be dry or sticky.
3. Abdomen; tight or flaccid.
4. Menopausal symptoms.
5. Hypertension due to liver/kidney disorders.
6. Liver and gallbladder disorders.
7. Edema, nephritis, pyelitis.
8. Diarrhea, dysuria, thirst.
9. Migraine.
10. Infectious summer disease.

Hoelen Five Herb Formula

Wu ling san

Polyporus	*Polyporus*	*Zhu ling*	4.5
Hoelen	*Poria*	*Fu ling*	4.5
Alisma	*Alismatis Rhizoma*	*Ze xie*	6.0
Atractylodes (white)	*Atractylodis Rhizoma*	*Bai shu*	4.5
Cinnamon Twigs	*Cinnamomi Ramulus*	*Gui zhi*	3.0

This is a harmonizing formula used for almost all water disorders in the body, and to treat conditions causing overall water metabolism disorders. The main symptoms are thirst, vomiting, dysuria, flushingup, palpitations, vertigo, anxiety, headache, abdominal pain, diarrhea, edema, and fever.

Functions:

Promotes yang, transforms qi, promotes diuresis, and dispels dampness.

Main Conformations:

Surface fever and interior water conformation, edema, decreased urine, diarrhea, water stagnation in the stomach with palpitations beneath the umbilicus, softness in the abdominal wall, vomiting of water, extreme thirst, vertigo, and headache.

Major Indications:

1. Pulse; floating and rapid, or sinking and soft.
2. Tongue; red with a thick coat, and can be either moist and swollen or dry and edematous.
3. Abdomen; soft and edematous (due to stagnant water) with water sounds in the stomach.
4. Water metabolism diseases.
5. Diarrhea and vomiting due to common cold.
6. Leukorrhea from cold/damp.
7. Diabetes.
8. Gastric disorders, including seasickness.
9. Migraine and recurrent headache.
10. Toxemia in pregnancy.
11. Overall bodyache.

References from the Classics:

Shang Han Lun, page 13. "A little water will settle the stomach and cure patients with greater yang disease when it manifests as dryness in the stomach following profuse perspiration induced by a sweating treatment, or as insomnia caused by anxiety and irritability and a desire to drink water. *Wu ling san* (Hoelen Five Herb Formula) is preferred for those cases with floating pulse, dysuria, mild fever, and (diabetic-like) thirst."

Shang Han Lun, page 14. "*Wu ling san* (Hoelen Five Herb Formula) is recommended (for patients) with a floating and rapid pulse, distress, and thirst after perspiring."

"*Wu ling san* (Hoelen Five Formula) is given for *shang han* (conditions) with perspiration and thirst."

"*Wu ling san* (Hoelen Five Formula) should be given for *chung feng* (*zhong feng*) conditions exhibiting a persistent, unrelieved fever over a period of six to seven days, along with symptoms of anxiety, intense thirst, and vomiting after ingestion of fluids."

Shang Han Lun, page 22. "Illness (fever, etc.), localized in the temporal area of the head, should be treated with the sweating method--*Gui zhi tang* (Cinnamon Combination) or *Ma huang tang* (Ma-huang Combination). Water applied to the temples represses the heat so that it cannot be dispersed. This results in severe anxiety, goose flesh (*cutis anserina*), and thirst, which ceases immediately upon drinking. This condition calls for *Wen ke san* (Meretix Formula); if a cure is not achieved, *Wu ling san* (Hoelen Five Herb Formula) is indicated. In cases with no heat conformation, but with cold inside accumulated in the chest, *Jie geng bai san* (Platycodon and Croton Formula) is given."

Shang Han Lun, page 24. "Greater yang disease which has been treated by a physician first with the sweating method, and then with the purgation method due to mistaken diagnosis of interior conformation, will exhibit relapsing fever and severe chills as a result of administering incorrect herbs, hardness beneath the heart with a sensation of tenderness on palpation, and a floating pulse. This condition should be treated with *Da huang huang lian xie xin tang* (Rhubarb, Coptis, and Scute Combination). Hardness beneath the heart, relapsing chills, and perspiration should be treated with *Fu zi xie hin tang* (Rhubarb and Aconite Combination). For patients in whom the hardness is not relieved by *Xie xin tang* (Pinellia Combination) and who experience thirst, dryness of the mouth, anxiety, and dysuria, *Wu ling san* (Hoelen Five Herb Combination) is indicated."

Shang Han Lun, page 57. "*Wu ling san* (Hoelen Five Herb Formula) is indicated for patients with vomiting, diarrhea, headache, fever, generalized aching, and thirst."

Chin Kuei Yao Lueh, page 88. "A thin individual who has palpitation beneath the navel, slobbering, and dizziness, has a water problem and needs *Wu ling san* (Hoelen Five Herb Formula)."

Chin Kuei Yao Lueh, page 94. "*Wu ling san* (Hoelen Five Herb Formula) stimulates urination and perspiration in patients with a floating pulse, oliguria, slight fever, and polydipsia."

"*Wu ling san* (Hoelen Five Herb Formula) treats thirst in patients who vomit water immediately after having drunk it. The condition is called water adversity."

Tang-kuei and Peony Formula

Dang gui shao yao san

Tang-kuei	*Angelicae Radix*	*Dang gui*	3.0
Peony	*Paeoniae Radix*	*Shao yao*	4.0
Hoelen	*Poria*	*Fu ling*	4.0
Atractylodes (white)	*Atractylodis Rhizoma*	*Bai shu*	4.0
Cnidium	*Cnidii Rhizoma (Ligustici Rhizoma)*	*Chuan xiong*	3.0
Alisma	*Alismatis Rhizoma*	*Ze xie*	4.0

This formula is used mainly for women with blood stagnation due to weakness. This includes postpartum weakness and lassitude in general, tendency to miscarriage, menstrual disorders, ob/gyn related urinary problems, and infertility. A patient suffering from nausea, vomiting, and loss of appetite should not take this formula.

Functions:

Tonifies blood and qi, activates blood, and promotes water metabolism.

Main Conformations:

Yin weakness conformation, chill conformation, irregular menstruation, prolonged menstrual flow, abnormal leukorrhea, lower abdominal and low back pain, abdominis rectus muscle spasm with softness of the abdominal wall, tinnitus, vertigo, heavy head, and anemia.

Major Indications:

1. Pulse; deep and weak.
2. Tongue; pale and puffy.
3. Abdomen; painful and soft with spasms of the rectus abdominis muscle, splashing sounds beneath the heart.
4. Postpartum weakness.
5. Menstrual and pregnancy disorders.
6. Cold body, especially the feet.
7. Tinnitus and vertigo.
8. Heaviness in head.
9. Pale skin and anemia.
10. Nephritis and cystitis.

References from the Classics:

Chin Kuei Yao Lueh, page 142. "*Dang gui shao yao san* (Tang-kuei and Peony Formula) helps pregnant women with abdominal cramping pain."

Chin Kuei Yao Lueh, page 157. "*Dang gui shao yao san* (Tang-kuei and Peony Formula) treats various women's abdominal problems."

Chapter 6

LIVER RELATED DISORDERS

The following formulas are arranged in order from the stronger and more aggressive to the more nutritive. The order is not meant as an absolute, but rather as a basic guide to how the formulas can be arranged for treatment.

These formulas basically fall within the yang stages of disease; that is tai yang, shao yang, and yang ming.

- Capillaris Combination
  (*Yin chen hao tang*)
- Bupleurum and Scute Combination
  (*Chai hu xian xiong tang*)
- Major Bupleurum Combination
  (*Da chai hu tang*)
- Minor Bupleurum Combination
  (*Xiao chai hu tang*)
- Bupleurum and Cinnamon Combination
  (*Chai hu gui zhi tang*)
- Bupleurum and Peony Formula
  (*Jia wei xiao yao san*)

- Bupleurum, Cinnamon, and Ginger Combination (*Chai hu gui zhi gan jiang tang)*
- Bupleurum and Dragon Bone Combination (*Chai hu jia long gu mu li tang*)
- Bupleurum and Hoelen Combination (*Chai long tang*)
- Peony and Licorice Combination (*Shao yao gan cao tang*)

Liver Related Disorder Symptoms

The following are basic disorders and indications commonly treated with the formulas in this section.

Cholecystitis

Symptoms: sudden fever and severe pain due to inflammation of the gallbladder.

Cholithiasis (Gallstones)

Symptoms: recurrent attacks of severe pain in the upper abdomen, upper abdominal discomfort, bloating, belching, and food intolerance. Foods high in animal fats can induce gallbladder attacks, which may result in jaundice, vomiting, and constipation.

Hepatitis

Symptoms: sudden onset of fever and flu-like symptoms such as general fatigue, anorexia, nausea, and abdominal pain. After two or three days, the icteric phase begins with the appearance of dark urine, jaundice, whiteness of the eyes, pressure and pain below the ribs due to an enlarged liver, and loss of appetite. Jaundice reaches a peak in about one to two weeks.

Formulas for Liver Related Disorders

Formula	Stage	Classification	Qi, Water Blood	Disorder	Patient Type
Capillaris C.	yang ming	diuretic	water blood	acute	strong
Bupleurum and Scute C.	tai yang/ shao yang	expectorant	qi	acute	strong
Major Bupleurum C.	tai yang/ yang ming	dual dissolving	qi	acute	strong
Minor Bupleurum C.	shao yang	harmonizing	qi	acute	medium
Bupleurum and Cinnamon C.	tai yang/ shao yang	dual dissolving	qi	acute/ chronic	medium/ weak
Bupleurum and Peony C.	shao yang	harmonizing	blood	acute	strong
Bupleurum, Cinnamon, and Ginger C.	shao yang	harmonizing	qi	chronic	medium/ weak
Bupleurum and Dragon Bone C.	shao yang	sedative	qi	chronic	weak
Bupleurum and Hoelen C.	shao yang	diuretic	water	chronic	weak
Licorice and Peony C.	shao yin/ jue yin	harmonizing	blood	chronic	weak

Capillaris Combination

Yin chen hao tang

Capillaris	*Artemisiae Capillaris Herba*	*Yin chen hao*	4.0
Gardenia	*Gardeniae Fructus*	*Zhi zi*	3.0
Rhubarb	*Rhei Rhizoma*	*Da huang*	1.0

Capillaris Combination is the same as the patent formula *Lidan Pian.* It is used for removing stagnant heat affecting the liver in a firm person with symptoms which include distention and discomfort in the upper abdomen and chest, nausea, thirst, dysuria, dark colored urine, and constipation.

Functions:

Clears heat, dispels dampness, and relieves jaundice.

Main Conformations:

Jaundice, mild fullness in the epigastrium with sensations of discomfort and irritability, abdominal fullness, constipation, extreme thirst, nausea, loss of appetite, head sweating, tongue coated yellow, and decreased urine.

Major Indications:

1. Pulse; deep, firm, and possibly wiry.
2. Tongue; yellow coat.
3. Abdomen; full and tight.
4. Jaundice, and hepatitis.
5. Nephritis.
6. Gingivitis.
7. Ophthalmic disorders.
8. Edema.
9. Uterine bleeding.

References from the Classics:

Shang Han Lun, page 40. "Sunlight yang disease with fever and perspiration will not result in yellowish discoloration of the skin (jaundice). However, cases with perspiration on the head and neck areas only, difficulty in urination, and a tendency to drink a lot of fluids will ultimately end in jaundice. *Yin chen hao tang* (Capillaris Combination) should be given."

Shang Han Lun, page 41. "*Shang han* (conditions) that have lasted seven to eight days, with a yellow-orange discoloration of the skin, dysuria, tendency toward constipation, and mild congestion in the abdomen should be treated mainly with *Yin chen hao tang* (Capillaris Combination)."

Chin Kuei Yao Lueh, page 113. "Chills and fever which cause anorexia, dizziness after eating, and discomfort in the heart and chest portend *ku tan* (cereal jaundice). The afflicted primarily needs *Yin chen hao tang* (Capillaris Combination)."

Bupleurum and Scute Combination

Chai hu xian xiong tang

Bupleurum	*Bupleuri Radix*	*Chai hu*	5.0
Pinellia	*Pinellia Tuber*	*Ban xia*	5.0
Scute	*Scutellariae Radix*	*Huang qin*	3.0
Ginseng	*Ginseng Radix*	*Ren shen*	2.0
Jujube	*Zizyphi Fructus*	*Da zao*	3.0
Ginger (fresh)	*Zingiberis Rhizoma*	*Sheng jiang*	3.0
Trichosanthes Seed	*Trichosanthis Semen*	*Gua lou ren*	3.0
Coptis	*Coptidis Rhizoma*	*Huang lian*	1.5
Licorice	*Glycyrrhizae Radix*	*Gan cao*	1.5

This formula is a mixture of *Xiao chai hu tang* (Minor Bupleurum Combination) and *Xiao xian xiong tang* (Minor Trichosanthes Combination), and is used for treating suppressed distention in the chest, chest pains due to coughing or deep breathing, viscous sputum, rapid respiration, recurrent chills and fever, bitter taste in the mouth, and loss of appetite.

Functions:

Dissolves phlegm, relieves chest distention, clears liver, and harmonizes stomach.

Major Indications:

1. Pulse; rapid and tight.

2. Tongue; yellow coat.

3. Abdomen; chronic water stagnancy in stomach.

4. Upper respiratory infections.

5. Common cold.

6. Hepatitis.

Major Bupleurum Combination

Da chai hu tang

Bupleurum	*Bupleuri Radix*	*Chai hu*	6.0
Scute	*Scutellariae Radix*	*Huang qin*	3.0
Pinellia	*Pinellia Tuber*	*Ban xia*	3.0
Ginger (fresh)	*Zingiberis Rhizoma*	*Sheng jiang*	4.0
Chih-shih	*Aurantii Fructus Immaturus*	*Zhi shi*	2.0
Peony	*Paeoniae Radix*	*Shao yao*	3.0
Rhubarb	*Rhei Rhizoma*	*Da huang*	1.0
Jujube	*Zizyphi Fructus*	*Da zao*	3.0

This formula should be taken only by those with an obese or strong constitution who have good *shen* (spirit), a strong sunken pulse, tightness beneath the heart, chest distention, pain in the chest, habitual constipation or diarrhea, vomiting, mental instability, and a tendency toward irritability.

Functions:

Soothes liver, clears heat, and relieves distention and constipation.

Main Conformation:

Obese or bony constitution, resistance and pain on palpation beneath the heart, thoracocostal distress, wide epigastric angle, alternating chills and fever, asthma, constipation, loss of appetite, nausea, vomiting, and yellow coated tongue.

Major Indications:

1. Pulse; deep, firm, slow, or rapid.
2. Tongue; yellow coat.
3. Abdomen; tense and firm.
4. Diabetes.
5. Liver and gallbladder disorders.
6. Habitual constipation or diarrhea.
7. Hypertension.
8. Gastritis and sour stomach.

9. Asthma.

10. Gastric distress, duodenal ulcer.

References from the Classics:

Shang Han Lun, page 17. "In cases of severe vomiting, with unrelieved stagnancy beneath the heart and distress in the chest, treatment with *Da chai hu tang* (Major Bupleurum Combination) may result in recovery after an episode of diarrhea."

Shang Han Lun, page 21. "For *shang han* (conditions) which persist for longer than ten days, and exhibit an accumulation of heat within the body together with alternating chills and fever (this is the fever type of lesser yang disease), *Da chai hu tang* (Major Bupleurum Combination) should be given."

Chin Kuei Yao Lueh, page 67. "Distention and aching beneath the heart due to firm evil should be purged with (*Da chai hu tang* (Major Bupleurum Combination), as the preferred drug."

Minor Bupleurum Combination

Xiao chai hu tang

Bupleurum	*Bupleuri Radix*	*Chai hu*	7.0
Scute	*Scutellariae Radix*	*Huang qin*	3.0
Pinellia	*Pinellia Tuber*	*Ban xia*	5.0
Ginseng	*Ginseng Radix*	*Ren shen*	3.0
Jujube	*Zizyphi Fructus*	*Da zao*	3.0
Licorice	*Glycyrrhizae Radix*	*Gan cao*	2.0
Ginger (fresh)	*Zingiberis Rhizoma*	*Sheng jiang*	4.0

Xiao chai hu tang (Minor Bupleurum Combination) is a harmonizing formula used for persons of average constitution experiencing symptoms associated with *shao yang* disease. The disease affects both the internal and external parts of the body, and will manifest primarily in the liver/gallbladder energy of the body. Symptoms may include chest distention, hardness beneath the heart, pain beneath the ribs and liver, loss of appetite, stress, vomiting, abdominal pain, bitter taste in mouth, and recurrent fever and chills.

Functions:

Soothes liver, cleanses gallbladder, and treats half-exterior/half-interior conformations.

Main Conformations:

Half-exterior/half-interior conformation, thoracocostal distress, obstruction and hardening beneath the heart, abdominal pain, chest pain, rigidity of the neck, deafness, bitter taste in the mouth, white tongue coat, alternating chills and fever, headache, and difficult urination

Main Indications:

1. Pulse; wiry/tight and either thin or quick.
2. Tongue; coated with white fur, possibly with a *ching* colored body and lateral edges without coating, and perhaps red dots on those edges.
3. Abdomen; full tightness in the upper abdomen and under the ribs, palpitation below the heart in the hypochondric area.
4. Common cold and upper respiratory infections with lingering fever and viscid sputum.
5. Liver and gallbladder disorders.
6. Thoracocostal and hypochondric fullness/obstruction.
7. Gastric disorders.
8. Infections of lymph glands, breasts, tonsils, lungs, uterus, and so forth.
9. Mental instability in children.

References from the Classics:

Shang Han Lun, page 16. "If the *shang han* [condition] persists for five to six days with alternating chills and fever, distress and fullness in the chest and ribs, silence with loss of appetite, disturbance in the heart with a tendency to vomit or disturbances in the chest without vomiting, thirst, abdominal aching, obstruction and stiffness beneath the ribs; or palpitations beneath the heart, dysuria, adypsia, mild generalized fever or cough, *Xiao chai hu tang* (Minor Bupleurum Combination) is indicated."

"For *shang han* conditions that have persisted for four to five days with somatic fever, severe chills, stiffness of the neck, fullness beneath the ribs, warm limbs, and thirst, *Xiao chai hu tang* (Minor Bupleurum Combination) is indicated."

Shang Han Lun, page 17. "Patients with a *shang han* condition with an obstructed, rough pulse, or superficial palpation and a tense pulse on deep touch having an acute abdominal ache should first take *Xiao jia zhong tang* (Minor Cinnamon and Peony Combination). If recovery is not complete, *Xiao chai hu tang* (Minor Bupleurum Combination) should be taken."

"Sometimes greater yang disease persists for more than ten days and moves slowly into the lesser yang stage. If it has been mistakenly treated with two or three purgations under the assumption that the disease has shifted to the sunlight yang stage, and four or five days later it still exhibits *Chai hu tang* (Bupleurum Combination) conformation, it should now be treated with *Xiao chai hu tang* (Minor Bupleurum Combination). In cases of severe vomiting after taking this combination, plus unrelieved stagnancy beneath the heart and distress in the chest, treatment with *Da chai hu tang* (Major Bupleurum Combination) may result in recovery after an episode of diarrhea."

Shang Han Lun, page 17-18. "If the *shang han* condition has persisted for about thirteen days with fullness between the chest and ribs, vomiting [lesser yang and *Chai hu tang* (Bupleurum Combination) conformation], tidal fever at sunset sunlight yang and *Da huang huang lian xie xin tang* (Rhubarb Combination) conformation and mild diarrhea, *Xiao chai hu tang* (Minor Bupleurum Combination) is recommended to relieve the surface symptoms, followed by *Chai hu mang xiao tang* (Bupleurum and Mirabilitum Combination)."

Shang Han Lun, page 22. "Women with *chung feng* conditions lasting seven to eight days, lingering chills and fever occurring at regular intervals (malaria-like symptoms), and amenorrhea and stagnancy of the blood should be treated primarily with *Xiao chai hu tang* (Minor Bupleurum Combination)."

Shang Han Lun, page 23. "*Shang han* conditions lasting five or six days with perspiration in the head area, mild chills, coldness of the hands and feet (two symptoms of lesser yin disease), congestion beneath the heart, loss of appetite (evidence of lesser yang disease), hard stools, and a small pulse may be treated with *Xiao chai hu tang* (Minor Bupleurum Combination). Recovery will occur when the bowel movements return to normal [an effect of Minor Bupleurum Combination]."

Shang Han Lun, page 38-39. "Sunlight yang disease, when present in combination with lesser yang disease, may exhibit hardness and congestion beneath the ribs, constipation (stagnancy in the lower jiao), vomiting (disharmony in the middle jiao), and white coating on the tongue (stagnancy in the upper jiao). *Xiao chai hu tang* (Minor Bupleurum Combination) is given to treat the upper jiao. When the upper jiao is normalized, the body fluids will then descend and circulate in the triple jiao, and the stomach will be harmonized. The problem is usually resolved following marked perspiration."

Shang Han Lun, page 39. "The *chung feng* condition of sunlight yang disease [is a combination of the three yang diseases]. The symptoms are tension (lesser yang), floating (greater yang), and large (sunlight yang) pulse, rapid respiration, abdominal congestion (sunlight yang conformation), pain beneath the ribs, and aching over the pericardium (lesser yang conformation), difficulty in breathing when pressure is applied to the abdomen, dryness of the nose, lack of perspiration (greater yang conformation), drowsiness, yellowish discoloration of the face and body (jaundice), difficulty in urination, tidal fever, frequent hiccoughs, and swelling around the ears (lesser yang conformation). If the swelling recedes, following acupuncture, but the outside symptoms linger for more than ten days with the floating pulse as before, then *Xiao chai hu tang* (Minor Bupleurum Combination) should be administered."

Shang Han Lun, page 44. "For patients with unrelieved manifestations of greater yang disease complicated by symptoms of lesser yang disease, including hardness and congestion beneath the ribs, retching, loss of appetite, alternating chills and fever, and a sinking and tight pulse, *Xiao chai hu tang* (Minor Bupleurum Combination) is recommended if the vomiting or purgation methods have been applied. If moxibustion, vomiting, or sweating methods have been used and there is delirium, it is of ominous import and indicates that the case has been mistreated. Now it is too late to institute the *chai hu ji* (bupleurum-containing formulas) as treatment."

Shang Han Lun, page 59. "*Xiao chai hu tang* (Minor Bupleurum Combination) is recommended for patients who have recovered from shang han conditions, but are having relapses of fever."

"*Chin Kuei Yao Lueh*, page 116. "*Xiao chai hu tang* (Minor Bupleurum Combination) treats various jaundice conditions with vomiting and abdominal aching."

Chin Kuei Yao Lueh, page 124. "A patient with vomiting and fever should be treated primarily with *Xiao chai hu tang* (Minor Bupleurum Combination)"

Chin Kuei Yao Lueh, page 146. "When a puerperal woman has depressive dizziness and a minute and weak pulse, vomits, has no appetite, passes hard stools, and perspires on the head only it is due to blood weakness and its consequent flushing of yang. The flushing always results in dizziness, and the patient will perspire profusely before the dizziness is relieved. Blood weakness and chills in the lower jiao leads to flushing of solitary yang and consequently sweating on the head. A puerperal woman needs to perspire because her exhaustion of yin and blood weakness leads to excessive yang. Sweating restores the balance of yin and yang. *Xiao chai hu tang* (Minor Bupleurum Combination) treats conformations with hard stools, vomiting, and loss of appetite."

Chin Kuei Yao Lueh, page 149. "When a puerperal woman has contracted wind evil because of exposure of her lower body during labor, and thus has limb distress, annoying fever and headache, she can be given *Xiao chai hu tang* (Minor Bupleurum Combination)."

Chin Kuei Yao Lueh, page 151. "A woman with 'contraction of winds' (i.e., heat in the liver) will have alternating seizures of chills and fever at fixed times. The seizures will last for seven to eight days and interrupt the menses. The fever invading the womb causes the blood to stagnate and produces malaria-type symptoms. Such a woman requires treatment with *Xiao chai hu tang* (Minor Bupleurum Combination)."

Bupleurum and Cinnamon Combination

Chai hu gui zhi tang

Bupleurum	*Bupleuri Radix*	*Chai hu*	5.0
Pinellia	*Pinellia Tuber*	*Ban xia*	4.0
Licorice	*Glycyrrhizae Radix*	*Gan cao*	1.5
Jujube	*Zizyphi Fructus*	*Da zao*	2.0
Cinnamon Twigs	*Cinnamomi Ramulus*	*Gui zhi*	2.5
Scute	*Scutellariae Radix*	*Huang qin*	2.0
Ginseng	*Ginseng Radix*	*Ren shen*	2.0
Peony	*Paeoniae Radix*	*Shao yao*	2.5
Ginger (dried)	*Zingiberis Siccatum Rhizoma*	*Gan jiang*	1.0

This formula is good for people with a somewhat delicate constitution who are experiencing extreme fatigue, gastrointestinal weakness, headache, heaviness in the head, neuralgia, fever and chills, distention beneath the heart, and lower abdominal pain. *Chai hu gui zhi tang* (Bupleurum and Cinnamon Combination) is a combination of *Xiao chai hu tang* (Minor Bupleurum Combination) and Gui zhi tang (Cinnamon Combination).

Functions:

Dispels wind, relieves exterior evil, harmonizes nutritive and protective qi, and harmonizes exterior and interior.

Main Conformations:

Greater yang and lesser yang conformation, neurotic behavior, mild vomiting, mild chills, pain in the joints, acute pain in the heart and abdomen, mild thoracocostal distress, and heavy head with headaches.

Major Indications:

1. Pulse; floating and weak.
2. Tongue; red and thick coat.

3. Abdomen; tense and distended--tenseness in the rectus abdominis muscles.
4. Respiratory infections.
5. Gastrointestinal disorders.
6. Chronic abdominal disorders.
7. Mental instability, nervous exhaustion.
8. Intercostal neuralgia, arthralgia.
9. "Wood over controlling earth" symptoms.
10. Female disorders.

References from the Classics:

Shang Han Lun, page 22. "*Shang han* conditions lasting six to seven days with fever, mild chills, persistent aching in the limbs, mild vomiting, and distention beneath the heart requires *Chai hu gui zhi tang (Bupleurum and Cinnamon Combination)*."

Chin Kuei Yao Lueh, page 71. "*Chai hu gui zhi tang* (Bupleurum and Cinnamon Combination) treats acute pain in the heart and abdomen."

Bupleurum and Peony Formula

Jia wei xiao yao san

Tang-kuei	*Angelicae Radix*	*Dang gui*	3.0
Peony	*Paeoniae Radix*	*Shao yao*	3.0
Gardenia	*Gardeniae Fructus*	*Zhi zi*	2.0
Atractylodes (white)	*Atractylodis Rhizoma*	*Bai shu*	3.0
Hoelen	*Poria*	*Fu ling*	3.0
Mentha	*Menthae Herba*	*Bo he*	1.0
Bupleurum	*Bupleuri Radix*	*Chai hu*	3.0
Moutan	*Moutan Radicis Cortex*	*Mu dan pi*	2.0
Ginger (dried)	*Zingiberis Siccatum Rhizoma*	*Gan jiang*	1.0
Licorice	*Glycyrrhizae Radix*	*Gan cao*	2.0

This is a harmonizing formula which has a broad spectrum of uses including gynecological disorders, aching of the arms and legs, mental instability, flushingup, dizziness, insomnia, thirst, and abdominal distention; all due to stagnant blood. The *Japanese Medical News* reports this formula to be the best remedy for cirrhosis, abdominal tenseness, thirst with persistent and bitter taste in the mouth, headache, turbid urine, and nosebleed.

Functions:

Soothes liver, removes liver qi stagnation, tonifies spleen and blood, purges excess fire, and regulates menstruation.

Main Conformations:

Facial flushing, afternoon flushingup sensation, mild thoracocostal distress, sweating, irritability, insomnia, headache, abnormal menstruation, and lassitude of the arms and legs.

Major Indications:

1. Pulse; tight and tense.
2. Tongue; purple or red dots.
3. Abdomen; tight.
4. Premenstrual syndrome.
5. Irregular menses and infertility.
6. Menopausal symptoms.
7. Leukorrhea.
8. Constipation.
9. Acute and chronic damp heat infections in the urogenital tract.

Bupleurum, Cinnamon, and Ginger Combination

Chai hu gui zhi gan jiang tang

Bupleurum	*Bupleuri Radix*	*Chai hu*	6.0
Cinnamon Twigs	*Cinnamomi Ramulus*	*Gui zhi*	3.0
Trichosanthes Roots	*Trichosanthis Radix*	*Gua lou gen*	3.0
Scute	*Scutellariae Radix*	*Huang qin*	3.0
Oyster Shell	*Ostreae Testa*	*Mu li*	3.0
Ginger (dried)	*Zingiberis Siccatum Rhizoma*	*Gan jiang*	2.0
Licorice	*Glycyrrhizae Radix*	*Gan cao*	2.0

This is a harmonizing formula which is used to treat people with delicate constitutions experiencing recurrent fever and chills, chest distention, palpitations, cold hands and feet, stress, insomnia, diarrhea, oliguria, thirst, and head sweats.

Functions:

Relieves exterior cold and clears interior heat.

Main Conformations:

Flushingup of qi, head sweats, extreme thirst, cardiac hyperfunction, thoracocostal distress with palpitation above the umbilicus, abdominal weakness, soft stools, decreased urine, chills around the waist and in the feet, and alternating chills and fever.

Major Indications:

1. Pulse; minute, thin, and rapid (quick).
2. Tongue; thick coat and pale.
3. Abdomen; weak.
4. Respiratory disorders.
5. Hepatitis, cholecystitis.
6. Blood diseases.
7. Gastric distention, peritonitis.
8. General deficient yang symptoms.

References from the Classics:

Shang Han Lun, page 23. "*Shang han*...that...exhibits fullness in the chest, dysuria, thirst without vomiting, perspiration in the head area, alternating chills and fever, and anxiety should be given *Chai hu gui zhi gan jiang tang* (Bupleurum, Cinnamon, and Ginger Combination)."

Chin Kuei Yao Lueh, page 30. "*Chai hu gui zhi gan jiang tang* (Bupleurum, Cinnamon, and Ginger Combination) treats malaria with chills and mild fever, or with chills and no fever."

Bupleurum and Dragon Bone Combination

Chai hu jia long gu mu li tang

Bupleurum	*Bupleuri Radix*	*Chai hu*	5.0
Hoelen	*Poria*	*Fu ling*	3.0
Pinellia	*Pinellia Tuber*	*Ban xia*	4.0
Rhubarb	*Rhei Rhizoma*	*Da huang*	1.0
Cinnamon Twigs	*Cinnamomi Ramulus*	*Gui zhi*	3.0
Scute	*Scutellariae Radix*	*Huang qin*	2.5
Jujube	*Zizyphi Fructus*	*Da zao*	2.5
Ginseng	*Ginseng Radix*	*Ren shen*	2.5
Ginger (fresh)	*Zingiberis Rhizoma*	*Sheng jiang*	2.5
Oyster Shell	*Ostreae Testa*	*Mu li*	2.5
Dragon Bone	*Draconis Os*	*Longgu*	0.0

This is a sedative formula which is used to relieve chest and subcardiac distention, palpitation at the abdomen, insomnia, irritability, fearfulness, unsteadiness, and tendencies toward mania and convulsions. When the yang of the liver is rising due to a deficiency of yin, this formula can help calm the mind and spirit.

Functions:

Harmonizes interior and exterior, pacifies the spirit, and induces calm.

Main Conformations:

Irritability, easily frightened, insomnia, delirium, chest distress, resistance and distention beneath the heart with palpitation above the umbilicus, constipation, decreased urine, sensation of lassitude, and edema.

Major indications:

1. Pulse; sinking and tight.
2. Tongue; slightly dry and white coat.
3. Abdomen; strong and palpitation above the umbilicus.
4. Anxiety.
5. Chest distress.
6. Palpitations near or above the umbilicus.

7. Hyperfunction of the heart.
8. Constipation.
9. Decreased urination.
10. Flushingup.
11. Neurosis.
12. Neurotic insomnia.

Reference from the Classics:

Shang Han Lun, page 18. "The patient still suffering from a *shang han* condition eight or nine days after treatment with the purgation method, and with a feeling of fullness in the chest, anxiety and nervousness, dysuria, delirium, heaviness of the body, and difficulty in turning should be treated mainly with *Chai hu jia long gu mu li tang* (Bupleurum and Dragon Bone Combination)."

Bupleurum and Hoelen Combination

Chai ling tang

Bupleurum	*Bupleuri Radix*	*Chai hu*	5.0
Pinellia	*Pinellia Tuber*	*Ban xia*	4.0
Scute	*Scutellariae Radix*	*Huang qin*	2.5
Ginseng	*Ginseng Radix*	*Ren shen*	2.5
Jujube	*Zizyphi Fructus*	*Da zao*	2.5
Ginger (fresh)	*Zingiberis Rhizoma*	*Sheng jiang*	4.0
Licorice	*Glycyrrhizae Radix*	*Gan cao*	2.0
Cinnamon Twigs	*Cinnamomi Ramulus*	*Gui zhi*	2.5
Polyporus	*Polyporus*	*Zhu ling*	2.5
Atractylodes (white)	*Atractylodis Rhizoma*	*Bai shu*	2.5
Hoelen	*Poria*	*Fu ling*	2.5
Alisma	*Alismatis Rhizoma*	*Ze xie*	4.0

Chai ling tang (Bupleurum and Hoelen Combination) is a mixture of *Xiao chai hu tang* (Minor Bupleurum Combination) and *Wu lin san* (Hoelen Five Formula). It is a harmonizing formula which is used to treat symptoms of the above mentioned formulas and is also used to treat thirst, edema, dysuria, and diarrhea. The conformation is that of water and/or blood mainly affecting the liver and kidney energies. This formula is safe to take over a long period of time.

Functions:

Dispels stagnant water, strengthens spleen, and harmonizes and relieves lesser yang disease.

Major Indications:

1. Pulse; tense and full or wiry.
2. Tongue; thick coat, but which may be dry.
3. Abdomen; tight or flaccid, depending upon water or qi conformation.
4. Menopausal symptoms.
5. Hypertension due to liver/kidney disorders.
6. Liver and gallbladder disorders.
7. Kidney disorders and edema.
8. Infectious summer diseases.

Peony and Licorice Combination

Shao yao gan cao tang

Peony	*Paeoniae Radix*	*Shao yao*	6.0
Licorice	*Glycyrrhizae Radix*	*Gan cao*	6.0

This is a harmonizing formula which is used to treat weakness in the legs and severe and painful muscle spasms in legs, stomach, intestines, bronchi, gallbladder, and ureters. The formula contains only peony and licorice. Peony dispels stagnant blood, relieves muscle spasms, and pacifies the liver. Licorice is an antispasmodic, analgesic, and detoxifier of blood.

Functions:

Relieves spasms and pain.

Main Conformations:

Pain in the interior, spasmodic pain in the arm and leg muscles, and spasm in the rectus abdominis muscles.

Major Indications:

1. Pulse; tight and/or wiry.
2. Tongue; purple with red dots on lateral sides and possible shaking.
3. Abdomen; tight, spasms in rectus abdominis muscles.
4. Spasms in waist and back.
5. Sciatica.
6. Rheumatic muscles, "50 year old" shoulders.
7. Intestinal cramps and colic.
8. Spasmodic cough and bronchial asthma.
9. Bladder, hemorrhoidal pain.
10. Weakness in legs.

Chapter 7

NEURASTHENIA AND INSOMNIA

The following formulas are arranged in order from the strongest to the more nutritive. The order is not an absolute but rather a basic guide to how formulas can be arranged for treatment.

During the shao yin stage (fifth stage) of disease when there is anxiety, the following could be considered:

- Bupleurum and Dragon Bone Combination
  (Chai hu jia long gu mu li tang)
- Bamboo and Hoelen Combination
  (Wen dan tang)
- Zizyphus Combination
  (Suan zao ren tang)
- Cinnabar Formula
  (Zhu sha an shen wan)
- Licorice and Jujube Combination
  (Gan mai da zhao tang)
- Ginseng and Zizyphus Combination
  (Tian wang bu xin dan)
- Ginseng and Longan Combination
  (Gui pi tang)

Neurasthenia and Insomnia Disorder Symptoms (Heart Related Disorders)

Neurasthenia

Symptoms: general fatigue, general aching and listlessness which are often associated with a neurotic state.

Insomnia

Symptoms: sleeplessness, restlessness, overactive thinking at night, and anxiety.

Formulas for Neurasthenia and Insomnia Disorders

Formula	Stage	Classification	Qi, Water Blood	Disorder	Patient Type
Bupleurum and Dragon Bone C.	shao yang	sedative	qi	chronic	weak
Bamboo and Hoelen C.	shao yin/ tai yin	harmonizing	qi/ water	chronic	weak
Zizyphus C.	tai yin/ shao yin	sedative	qi/ blood	chronic	weak
Cinnabar Sedative C.	shao yin	sedative	qi/ blood	chronic	weak
Licorice and Jujube C.	shao yin	sedative	qi	chronic	weak
Ginseng and Zizyphus C.	shao yin	tonic	qi/ blood	chronic	weak
Ginseng and Longan C.	tai yin/ shao yin	blood	blood	chronic	weak

Bupleurum and Dragon Bone Combination

Chai hu jia long gu mu li tang

Bupleurum	*Bupleuri Radix*	*Chai hu*	5.0
Hoelen	*Poria*	*Fu ling*	3.0
Pinellia	*Pinellia Tuber*	*Ban xia*	4.0
Rhubarb	*Rhei Rhizoma*	*Da huang*	1.0
Cinnamon Twigs	*Cinnamomi Ramulus*	*Gui zhi*	3.0
Scute	*Scutellariae Radix*	*Huang qin*	2.5
Jujube	*Zizyphi Fructus*	*Da zao*	2.0
Ginseng	*Ginseng Radix*	*Ren shen*	2.5
Ginger (fresh)	*Zingiberis Rhizoma*	*Sheng jiang*	2.5
Oyster Shell	*Ostreae Testa*	*Mu li*	2.5
Dragon Bone	*Draconis Os*	*Long gu*	2.5

This ia a harmonizing-sedative formula which is used for many psycho-neurological symptoms associated with agitation, as well as feelings of stagnation in the chest and upper abdomen; it is used to treat true or false heat in the liver which in turn causes mental restlessness. This formula is effective in harmonizing the exterior and interior of the body, and has a sedating effect on the mind. *Chai hu jia long gu mu li tang* (Bupleurum and Dragon Bone Combination) is also a diuretic. The type of person this formula is used for is yin weak and yang strong; a typical type-A personality. This formula has proven very effective in the treatment of hyperactive children with strong constitutions. If the child has a weak constitution, *Gui zhi jia long gu mu li tang* (Cinnamon and Dragon Bone Combination) may be used instead.

Functions:

Harmonizes interior and exterior, pacifies the spirit, and induces calm.

Main Conformations:

Irritable, easily frightened, insomniac, delirious, chest distress, resistance and distention beneath the heart with palpitation above the umbilicus, constipation, decreased urine, sensation of lassitude, and edema.

Major Indications:

1. Pulse; tense, rapid, and wiry.
2. Tongue; purple or red, possibly with red dots on the lateral edges, a red tip, and/or quivering.
3. Abdomen; tight with resistance and distention in the hypochondriac area and palpitations above the umbilicus.
4. Insomnia, hysteria, delirium, and neurosis.
5. Constipation and/or edema.
6. Hypertension.
7. Heart disease.
8. Epilepsy.
9. Neurotic impotence/menopausal disorders.

References from the Classics:

Shang Han Lun, page 18. "The patient who continues to suffer from a *shang han* (condition) eight to nine days after treatment with the purgation method, (and has a feeling of) fullness in the chest, anxiety and nervousness, dysuria, delirium, heaviness of the body, and difficulty in turning should be treated with *Chai hu jia long gu mu li tang* (Bupleurum and Dragonbone Combination)."

Bamboo and Hoelen Combination

Wen dan tang

Citrus	*Citri Leiocarpae Exocarpium*	*Chen pi*	2.5
Hoelen	*Poria*	*Fu ling*	6.0
Pinellia	*Pinellia Tuber*	*Ban xia*	6.0
Chih-shih	*Aurantii Fructus Immaturus*	*Zhi shi*	1.5
Bamboo (shavings)	*Bambusae Caulis Et Taeniis*	*Zhu ru*	2.0
Ginger (fresh)	*Zingiberis Rhizoma*	*Sheng jiang*	3.0
Licorice	*Glycyrrhizae Radix*	*Gan cao*	1.0
Coptis	*Coptidis Rhizoma*	*Huang lian*	1.0
Zizyphus	*Zizyphi Spinosi Semen*	*Suan zao ren*	3.0

This is a harmonizing formula which is used for persons with water stagnation in the middle jiao causing gastric distress and mental instability. The person will be of weak conformation and have a "spleen" body type. This formula is associated with a diagnostic configuration of heat in the middle jiao affecting the upper jiao.

Functions:

Harmonizes stomach, subdues ascending qi, relieves vomiting, and dispels excess fluid.

Main Conformations:

Weak constitution, weakness and pain after illness, neurotic hypersensitivity, insomnia and nightmares, spontaneous sweating and night sweats, obstruction beneath the heart with water stagnation in the stomach, and abdominal weakness.

Major Indications:

1. Pulse; weak and slippery.
2. Tongue; greasy coat, pale, and possibly swollen.
3. Abdomen; water stagnancy, weak, and water sounds upon palpation of the upper abdomen.
4. Insomnia and palpitations.
5. Gastric disorders.
6. Loss of appetite.
7. Nightmares and easily frightened.
8. Spontaneous sweating and night sweats.

Zizyphus Combination

Suan zao ren tang

Zizyphus	*Zizyphi Spinosi Semen*	*Suan zao ren*	10.0
Hoelen	*Poria*	*Fu ling*	5.0
Cnidium	*Cnidii Rhizoma (Ligustici Rhizoma)*	*Chuan xiong*	3.0
Licorice	*Glycyrrhizae Radix*	*Gan cao*	1.0
Anemarrhena	*Anemarrhenae Rhizoma*	*Zhi mu*	3.0

This combination is also available in a patent formula: *Tabelle Suan Zao Ren Tang*. Is is a sedative formula which is used to treat deficiency in heart and liver yin and blood in persons who are experiencing weakness, fatigue, insomnia, and nervous exhaustion. This person will have a delicate constitution.

Functions:

Relieves irritability and pacifies spirit.

Main Conformations:

Cardiac hyperfunction, insomnia or somnolence, amnesia, terror, nightmares, night sweats, abdominal weakness, and fatigue.

Major Indications:

1. Pulse; weak, thready, and rapid.
2. Tongue; pale or red, possibly red tipped.
3. Abdomen; weak.
4. Nervous exhaustion.
5. Insomnia and nightmares.
6. Night sweats.
7. Vertigo.
8. Amnesia.
9. Flushingup.
10. Tight tendons and muscles.
11. Rapid heart palpitations.

References from the Classics:

Chin Kuei Yao Lueh, page 45. "*Suan zao ren tang* (Zizyphus Combination) is primarily used to treat weakness, fatigue, and annoyance due to weakness which causes insomnia."

Cinnabar Sedative Formula

Zhu sha an shen wan

Coptis	*Coptidis Rhizoma*	*Huang lian*	4.5
Cinnabar	*Cinnabaris*	*Zhu sha*	3.0
Tang-kuei	*Angelicae Radix*	*Dang gui*	3.0
Rehmannia (raw)	*Rehmanniae Radix*	*Sheng di huang*	3.0
Licorice	*Glycyrrhizae Radix*	*Gan cao*	1.5

This is a sedative formula which is used to treat strong or weak persons with internal heat, deficient heart yin causing emotional instability, insomnia, nightmares, and stress causing fever in the chest.

Functions:

Calms the heart and spirit

Major Indications:

1. Pulse; thready, weak, and rapid.
2. Tongue; red, no coat or, in some cases, red dots all over the tongue body.
3. Abdomen; tight.
4. Insomnia.
5. Palpitations.
6. Neurasthenia.
7. Amnesia.

Licorice and Jujube Combination

Gan mai da zao tang

Licorice	*Glycyrrhizae Radix*	*Gan cao*	5.0
Wheat	*Tritici Fructus*	*Fu xiao mai*	20.0
Jujube	*Zizyphi Fructus*	*Da zao*	6.0

This is a sedating formula which relaxes both the mind and the muscles of the body. The patient will have a deficient constitution and can be either lean and wiry or flabby and heavy, but will have a general lack of muscle tone and a susceptibility to pain.

Functions:

Nourishes the heart, pacifies the spirit, and relieves acute symptoms.

Main Conformations:

Despair and crying, excitability, insomnia, coma, hysteria, frequent yawning, general spasmodic muscles, and convulsions in the rectus abdominis muscles.

Major Indications:

1. Pulse; generally deep and deficient, although on a superficial level it can be rapid and tight/wiry.
2. Tongue; pale, quivering, possibly red tipped, and curving to one side.
3. Abdomen; tight with spasms.
4. Hysteria, neuroses.
5. Nervous exhaustion.
6. Insomnia, sleepwalking, and night crying.
7. Epilepsy, chorea.
8. Gastrointestinal and uterine cramping and spasms.
9. Spasmodic cough.
10. Muscle spasms.

References from the Classics:

Chin Kuei Yao Lueh, page 152-153. "A woman with visceral irritation (hysteria) tends to grieve and cry as though possessed by a spirit. She also yawns frequently. She needs *Gan mai da zao tang* (Licorice and Jujube Combination).... This formula supplements splenic qi."

Ginseng and Zizyphus Formula

Tian wang bu xin dan

Rehmannia (raw)	*Rehmanniae Radix*	*Sheng di huang*	1.2
Ginseng	*Ginseng Radix*	*Ren shen*	1.2
Scrophularia	*Scrophulariae Radix*	*Xuan shen*	1.2
Salvia	*Salviae Miltiorrhziae Radix*	*Dan shen*	1.2
Hoelen	*Poria*	*Fu ling*	1.2
Platycodon	*Platycodi Radix*	*Jie geng*	1.2
Polygala	*Polygalae Radix*	*Yuan zhi*	1.2
Biota	*Biotae Semen*	*Bo zi ren*	1.2
Asparagus	*Asparagi Radix*	*Tian men tung*	1.2
Ophiopogon	*Ophiopogonis Tuber*	*Mai men tong*	1.2
Tang-kuei	*Angelicae Radix*	*Dang gui*	1.2
Schizandra	*Schizandrae Fructus*	*Wu wei zi*	1.2
Acorus	*Acori Rhizoma*	*Shi chang pu*	1.2
Cinnabar	*Cinnabaris*	*Zhu sha*	1.2
Zizyphus	*Zizyphi Spinosi Semen*	*Suan zao ren*	1.2
Coptis	*Coptidis Rhizoma*	*Huang lian*	1.2

Tian wang bu xin dan (Ginseng and Zizyphus Combination) is used for weak persons with deficient heart yin since it slowly nourishes the yin of the upper burner. It can also be used for hyperactivity in children who have weak constitutions. The formula not only acts on the heart, but also tonifies kidney energy so that the kidneys better control the heart. Many conditions that utilize this formula manifest symptoms of heat above and deficiency below.

Functions:

Nourishes yin, supplements blood, nourishes, heart and pacifies spirit.

Major Indications:

1. Pulse; thready, weak, rapid, and tense.
2. Tongue; red, no coat, or possibly red tip.
3. Abdomen; flaccid, with strong pulsation of the abdominal aorta on the right side of the midline.

4. Thin in chest and face.
5. Reddish complexion.
6. Emotional instability and amnesia.
7. Palpitations and insomnia.
8. Constipation.
9. Nocturnal emissions and night sweats.

Contraindications:

Patients with gastrointestinal weakness, and moist, tenacious sputum should avoid taking this formula.

Ginseng and Longan Combination

Gui pi tang

Astragalus	*Astragali Radix*	*Huang qi*	2.0
Ginseng	*Ginseng Radix*	*Ren shen*	3.0
Hoelen	*Poria*	*Fu ling*	3.0
Atractylodes (white)	*Atractylodis Rhizoma*	*Bai shu*	3.0
Zizyphus	*Zizyphi Spinosi Semen*	*Suan zao ren*	3.0
Longan	*Longanae Arillus*	*Long yan rou*	3.0
Tang-kuei	*Angelicae Radix*	*Dang gui*	2.0
Ginger (dried)	*Zingiberis Siccatum Rhizoma*	*Gan jiang*	1.0
Jujube	*Zizyphi Fructus*	*Da zao*	1.0
Polygala	*Polygalae Radix*	*Yuan zhi*	1.0
Licorice	*Glycyrrhizae Radix*	*Gan cao*	1.0
Saussurea	*Saussureae Radix*	*Mu xiang*	1.0

This is a blood building and moving formula which is generally used for women with spleen/heart imbalance (i.e., deficient spleen robbing heart yin) affecting the qi and blood; this causes gastrointestinal weakness, menstrual irregularities, and insomnia. It can also be used for an acute or recent loss of blood which may cause overall debility. The person for whom this formula is intended will have a weak constitution.

Functions:

Tonifies qi, strengthens spleen, supplements blood, nourishes heart, and pacifies the spirit.

Main Conformations:

Cardiac hyperfunction, facial pallor, neurosis, insomnia, amnesia, coughing of blood, abdominal laxity, menstrual irregularity, hemorrhage including intestinal and uterine, urinary bleeding, and fatigue.

Major Indications:

1. Pulse; deep, thin and weak, or possibly thready and/or empty.
2. Tongue; pale, no coat, and possibly flabby.
3. Abdomen; flabby and weak.
4. Irregular menses and postpartum weakness.
5. Amnesia, insomnia, fatigue, and nervous exhaustion.
6. Bleeding (due to *xu* spleen qi) and hemorrhage.
7. Talk about self excessively and obsessed with self.
8. Anemia, pale complexion, and anorexia.
9. Flabby and no muscle tone.
10. Excess perspiration and night sweats.
11. Leukemia, and uterine carcinoma.
12. Endometritis and genital itching.
13. Impotence and chronic gonorrhea.

Chapter 8

JOINT AND NERVE DISORDERS

The following formulas are arranged in order from the stronger and more aggressive to the more nutritive. The order is not meant as an absolute, but rather as a basic guide to how the formulas can be arranged for treatment.

During the tai yang (first) stage of nerve and joint disorders, the following formulas should be considered:

- Coptis and Scute Combination
  (*Huang lian jie du tang*)
- Pueraria Combination
  (*Ge gen tang*)
- Atractylodes Combination
  (*Yue bi jia zhu tang*)
- Clematis and Carthamus Formula
  (*Shu jin li an san*)
- Coix Combination
  (*Yi yi ren tang*)
- Cinnamon and Atractylodes Combination
  (*Gui zhi jia ling shu fu tang*)

During the shao yang (second) stage of nerve and joint disorders, the following formulas should be considered:

- Cinnamon and Hoelen Formula
  (*Gui zhi fu ling wan*)

- Hoelen Five Herb Formula
  (*Wu ling san*)

- Bupleurum and Gardenia Formula
  (*Chai hu shu san*)

During the yang ming (third stage) of nerve and joint disorders, the following should be considered:

- Persica and Rhubarb Combination
  (*Tao he cheng qi tang*)

During the tai yin (fourth) stage of nerve and joint disorders, the following should be considered:

- Clematis and Stephania Combination
  (*Shu jing huo xue tang*)

- Ginseng and Ginger Combination
  (*Li zhong tang*)

- Tang-kuei, Evodia and Ginger Combination
  (*Dang gui si ni jia wu zhu yu sheng jiang tang*)

- Ginseng and Tang-kuei Ten Combination
  (*Shi quan da bu tang*)

During the shao yin and jue yin (fifth and sixth) stages of nerve and joint disorders, the following should be considered:

- Rehmannia Eight Formula
  (*Ba wei di huang wan*)

- Ma-huang, Aconite, and Asarum Combination
  (*Ma huang xi xin fu zi tang*)

Joint and Nerve Disorder Symptoms

The following is a list of basic disorders and indications commonly treated with the formulas in this section.

Arthrosis Deformans of the Knee

Symptoms: joint aches when exercising or lifting heavy objects, lessening of flexibility and movement of the knee joint, and mild contractions and swelling of the synovial bursa.

Facial Nerve Paralysis (Bell's Palsy)

Symptoms: distorted facial appearance with one side of the face and its mimic muscles paralyzed, frontal folds disappear, eyes and mouth unable to close properly, loss of taste sense, and, at times, deafness may result.

Migraine

Symptoms: throbbing headaches caused by cerebral meningeal, and extracranial, arterial vasoconstriction followed by dilation and distention of cranial vessels. Characteristically, the headache is accompanied by gastrointestinal or visual symptoms (nausea, vomiting, impaired vision, sensitivity to light, blindness in half of the visual field, or blurred vision.

Myelitis

Symptoms: back pain, girdle sensation, hyperesthesia, formication, anesthesia, motor disturbance, paralysis, increased reflexes, paralysis of sphincters, decubitus ulcers, and, in later stages, spasmodic contraction of paralyzed limbs.

Spondylosis Deformans (Osteoarthritis)

Symptoms: deformation on the edge of the vertebra, especially the superior-anterior and inferior edges, and involvement of the intervertebral joint and spinous process.

Formulas for Joint and Nerve Disorders

Formula	Stage	Classification	Qi, Water Blood	Disorder	Patient Type
Coptis Scute C.	tai yang/ shao yang	fire purging	qi	acute	strong
Pueraria C.	tai yang	sudorific	qi	acute	medium
Atractylodes C.	tai yang/ tai yin	diuretic	water	acute	strong
Clematis and Carthamus C.	tai yang/ jue yin	carminative	qi/ blood	chronic/ acute	strong/ weak
Coix C.	tai yang/ jue yin	diuretic	water/ blood	chronic	strong
Cinnamon and Atractylodes C.	tai yang	sudorific	qi	chronic	weak
Cinnamon and Hoelen C.	shao yang	blood	qi/ blood	chronic	weak
Hoelen Five C.	shao yang/ shao yin	diuretic	water	chronic	weak
Bupleurum and Gardenia C.	shao yang/ jue yin	blood	blood/ qi	chronic	strong
Persica and Rhubarb C.	yang ming	blood	blood	chronic	strong
Clematis and Stephania C.	tai yin/ jue yin	blood	blood/ water	chronic	medium
Ginseng and Ginger C.	tai yin	chill dispelling	water	acute/ chronic	weak
Ma-huang, Aconite, and Asarum C.	shao yin/ tai yang	sudorific	qi	chronic	weak
Tang-kuei Evodia and Ginger C.	tai yin	chill dispelling	qi blood	chronic	weak
Ginseng and Tang-kuei Ten C.	tai yin/ jue yin	tonic	qi blood	chronic	weak
Rehmannia Eight C.	shao yin	tonic	water/ chronic	blood	weak

Coptis and Scute Combination

Huang lian jie du tang

Scute	*Scutellariae Radix*	*Huang qin*	3.0
Coptis	*Coptidis Rhizoma*	*Huang lian*	1.5
Gardenia	*Gardeniae Fructus*	*Zhi zi*	2.0
Phellodendron	*Phellodendri Cortex*	*Huang bo*	1.5

This is a heat clearing formula which is used to treat strong persons who have true heat signs causing inflammation, anxiety, bleeding, and overall congestion. It can address heat in any organ system, but mainly is used in liver fire conditions; it brings down heat, moves blood, and detoxifies.

Functions:

Clears heat, purges fire, arrests bleeding, and relieves irritability.

Main Conformations:

Yang strong conformation, cardiac hyperfunction, restlessness and insomnia, spitting and vomiting blood, facial reddening, chest discomfort with sensation of resistance beneath the heart, forceful abdomen, melena in stools (stools resembling tar in appearance), and red urine.

Major Indications:

1. Pulse: forceful, deep, and rapid.
2. Tongue: red and possible yellow coated.
3. Abdomen: strong and tight.
4. Hypertension, anxiety
5. Constipation.
6. Bleeding disorders (due to true heat).
7. Insomnia.
8. Resistance beneath the heart and palpitations.
9. Cerebral hemorrhage.
10. Herpes and urticaria.
11. Joint and nerve disorders.

Pueraria Combination

Ge gen tang

Pueraria	*Puerariae Radix*	*Ge gen*	8.0
Ma-huang	*Ephedrae Herba*	*Ma huang*	4.0
Cinnamon	*Cinnamomi Ramulus*	*Gui zhi*	3.0
Peony	*Paeoniae Radix*	*Shao yao*	3.0
Ginger (dried)	*Zingiberis Siccatum Rhizoma*	*Gan jiang*	1.0
Jujube	*Zizyphi Fructus*	*Da zao*	4.0
Licorice	*Glycyrrhizae Radix*	*Gan cao*	2.0

Pueraria Combination is used for treating *tai yang* disease in average and strong persons with severe muscle spasms, stiffness, common cold (febrile or afebrile), and anhidrosis.

Functions:

Relieves external symptoms and muscle ache, promotes blood circulation, and alleviates pain.

Main Conformations:

Yang-firm conformation, stiffness and spasms in the neck and upper back, general aching, headaches, flushingup, anhidrosis, diarrhea, and painful urination.

Major Indications:

1. Pulse; floating, strong, rapid, and tense.

2. Tongue; thin, white coated, and possibly moist and/or red.

3. Abdomen; tight.

4. Muscular aches and pains, neuralgia.

5. Common cold, and upper respiratory infections.

6. Asthma.

7. Skin diseases.

8. Mastitis and lymphadenitis.

References from the Classics:

Shang Han Lun, page 9. "Greater yang disease in which there is a sensation of stiffness and heaviness in the neck and back, and mild chills (anemophobia) but no perspiration should be given *Ge gen tang* (Pueraria Combination)."

Shang Han Lun, page 9. "*Ge gen tang* (Pueraria Combination) is given to patients experiencing diarrhea as a complication of greater and sunlight yang diseases."

Chin Kuei Yao Lueh, page 12. "Greater yang disease with anhidrosis, oliguria, flushing of qi towards the chest, lockjaw, and a tendency to have strong convulsions should be treated with *Ge gen tang* (Pueraria Combination)."

Atractylodes Combination

Yue bi qia zhu tang

Ma-huang	*Ephedrae Herba*	*Ma huang*	6.0
Gypsum	*Gypsum Fibrosum*	*Shi gao*	8.0
Jujube	*Zizyphi Fructus*	*Da zao*	3.0
Licorice	*Glycyrrhizae Radix*	*Gan cao*	2.0
Atractylodes (white)	*Atractylodis Rhizoma*	*Bai shu*	4.0
Ginger (fresh)	*Zingiberis Rhizoma*	*Sheng jiang*	3.0

This formula is used to treat kidney yang deficient persons with lower limb edema, rheumatism, acute bursitis, and water stagnancy in the lower *jiao*.

Functions:

Dispels stagnant water and reduces swelling.

Main Conformations:

Edema, extreme thirst, spontaneous sweating, hard stools, decreased urine, tearing eyes, and pain in the hands and feet.

Major Indications:

1. Pulse; deep and may be wiry.
2. Tongue; red with dry or sticky coat.
3. Abdomen; tight.
4. Arthritis, rheumatism pain in hands and feet.
5. Polyps.
6. Chillphobia.
7. Edema.
8. Kidney disorders.
9. Skin disorders due to water toxins.
10. Gout with chills, moisture, and wind symptoms.
11. Acute pain in the joints.
12. Weak and aching feet.

References from the Classics:

Chin Kuei Yao Lueh, page 39. "*Yue bi jia zhu tang* (Atractylodes Combination) treats muscle exhaustion, which, in the presence of fever, exhibits loss of body fluids, enlarged pores, muscle looseness, and profuse sweating. It also alleviates severe wind and weakness of the lower jiao and feet."

Chin Kuei Yao Lueh, page 99. "Interior water-yellow swelling all over the body including the face and eyes, submerged pulse, and oliguria primarily requires *Yue bi jia zhu tang* (Atractylodes Combination). However, polyuria, which is causing loss of fluids and hence thirst, contraindicates this formula."

Chin Kuei Yao Lueh, page 105. "A skin water disease can be treated primarily with *Yue bi jia zhu tang* (Atractylodes Combination)..."

Clemetis and Carthamus Formula

Shu jin li an san

Siler	*Ledebouriellae Radix*	*Fang feng*	1.2
Chiang-huo	*Notopterygii Rhizoma*	*Qiang huo*	1.2
Tu-huo	*Angelicae Tuhuo Radix*	*Du huo*	1.2
Cnidium	*Cnidii Rhizoma (Ligustici Rhizoma)*	*Chuan xiong*	1.2
Hoelen	*Poria*	*Fu-ling*	1.2
Angelica	*Angelicae Dahuricae Radix*	*Bai zhi*	1.2
Rehmannia	*Rehmanniae Radix*	*Di huang*	1.2
Atractylodes (white)	*Atractylodis Rhizoma*	*Bai shu*	1.2
Carthamus	*Carthami Flos*	*Hong hua*	1.2
Persica	*Persicae Semen*	*Tao ren*	1.2
Arisaema	*Arisaematis Rhizoma*	*Tian nan xing*	1.2
Citrus	*Citri Leiocarpae Exocarpium*	*Chen pi*	1.2
Pinellia	*Pinellia Tuber*	*Ban xia*	1.2
Achyranthes	*Achyranthis Radix*	*Niu xi*	1.2
Clematis	*Clematidis Radix*	*Wei ling xian*	1.2
Stephania	*Aristolochiae Fangchi Radix*	*Fang ji*	1.2
Chaenomeles	*Chaenomelis Fructus*	*Mu gua*	1.2
Forsythia	*Forsythiae Fructus*	*Lian qiao*	1.2
Aconite (processed)	*Aconiti Carmichaelii Praeparata Radix*	*Fu zi*	0.5-1.0
Akebia	*Akebiae Caulis*	*Mu tong*	1.2
Licorice	*Glycyrrhizae Radix*	*Gan cao*	1.2
Bamboo (shavings)	*Bambusae Caulis Et Taeniis*	*Zhu ru*	1.2
Gentiana	*Gentianae Scabrae Radix*	*Long dan*	1.2
Scute	*Scutellariae Radix*	*Huang qin*	1.2
Atractylodes (red)	*Atractylodis Lanceae Rhizoma*	*Cang shu*	1.2

This formula has twenty-five different herbs and can be used for any type of arthritis due to stagnant qi or blood. Not only does it relieve stagnation, but it also tonifies and has an analgesic affect on the body.

Functions:

Dispels wind, cold dampness and heat, and activates blood and the meridians.

Major Indications:

1. Pulse; tight and wiry.
2. Abdomen; tight.
3. Tongue; dark red.
4. Acute or chronic arthritis (especially rheumatoid).
5. Palsy.
6. Monoplegia.
7. Severe pain in the limbs and joints.

Coix Combination

Yi yi ren tang

Ma-huang	*Ephedrae Herba*	*Ma huang*	4.0
Tang-kuei	*Angelicae Radix*	*Dang gui*	4.0
Coix	*Coicis Semen*	*Yi yi ren*	8.0
Atractylodes (white)	*Atractylodis Rhizoma*	*Bai shu*	4.0
Cinnamon Twigs	*Cinnamomi Ramulus*	*Gui zhi*	3.0
Peony	*Paeoniae Radix*	*Shao yao*	3.0
Licorice	*Glycyrrhizae Radix*	*Gan cao*	2.0

This formula is very effective in treating rheumatism and arthritis due to heat, stagnant blood, and/or water accumulation. It promotes the circulation of stagnant blood, dispels excess fluid, and relieves muscle tension. It is said to cure muscle spasms, aching, numbness, swelling and slackness of the limbs. It is also effective in treating cysts on fleshy areas of the body due to water or blood stagnation.

Functions:

Dispels wind and dampness, activates blood, and relieves numbness and pain.

Main Conformations:

Sensation of heat in the joints, pain in the arms and legs, beriberi, and impaired movement or paralysis of the legs

Major Indications:

1. Pulse; tight and wiry.
2. Tongue; red or purple.
3. Abdomen; swollen, with spasms and pain.
4. Feverish sensation.
5. Pain and spasms in the arms and legs.
6. Rheumatism and arthritis.
7. Nephritis and pulmonary edema.
8. Paralysis.
9. Overall pain and swelling of the joints.
10. Chill and numbness in any joint.

Cinnamon and Atractylodes Combination

Gui zhi jia ling shu fu tang

Cinnamon	*Cinnamomi Ramulus*	*Gui zhi*	3.0
Peony	*Paeoniae Radix*	*Shao yao*	3.0
Jujube	*Zizyphi Fructus*	*Da zao*	3.0
Ginger (fresh)	*Zingiberis Rhizoma*	*Sheng jiang*	3.0
Licorice	*Glycyrrhizae Radix*	*Gan cao*	1.5
Hoelen	*Poria*	*Fu Ling*	5.0
Atractylodes (white)	*Atractylodis Rhizoma*	*Bai shu*	5.0
Aconite (processed)	*Aconiti Carmichaelii Praeparata Radix*	*Fu zi*	0.5-1.0

This formula can be used to treat weak persons who have delicate stomachs and water toxin.

Functions:

Dispels wind and cold, strengthens spleen, and removes dampness.

Major Indications:

1. Pulse; weak, slow, and possibly knotted.
2. Tongue; pale.
3. Abdomen; weak.
4. Spasms in arms and legs.
5. Neuralgia, arthralgia, and arthritis.
6. Dysuria.
7. Headache.
8. Severe chills.
9. Apoplexy.

Cinnamon and Hoelen Formula

Gui zhi fu ling wan

Cinnamon Twigs	*Cinnamomi Ramulus*	*Gui zhi*	4.0
Hoelen	*Poria*	*Fu ling*	4.0
Persica	*Persicae Semen*	*Tao ren*	4.0
Peony	*Paeoniae Radix*	*Shao yao*	4.0
Moutan	*Moutan Radicis Cortex*	*Mu dan pi*	4.0

This formula is used to treat joint, nerve and gynecological disorders due to stagnant blood; it is used only for strong conformations whose symptoms include flushed face, protruding abdomen, resistant pressing pain at the umbilicus, shoulder stiffness, and chills in the feet.

Functions:

Dispels stagnant blood and lumps in the abdomen.

Main Conformations:

Blood stagnation in the face and lips, cardiac hyperfunction, spasm in the left rectus abdominis muscle, lumps in lower abdomen (weak pain on pressure), lower abdominal and low back pain, melena stool (evacuation resembling tar), and menstrual irregularity

Major Indications:

1. Pulse; tense, sunken, and slow.

2. Tongue; purple and *ching.*
3. Abdomen; tight with lumps and spasms.
4. Gynecological diseases due to blood stagnation.
5. Arthritis, rheumatism, and neuralgia.
6. Skin diseases.
7. Lumbago and shoulder pain.
8. Headaches and vertigo.
9. Eye disorders.
10. Neuropathy; nervousness, neurosis, and hysteria.

References from the Classics:

Chin Kuei Yao Lueh, page 141. "Movement above the navel and sudden incessant uterine bleeding three months after the cessation of menses indicates the presence of a tumor. However, movement in the sixth month with regular menses in the first three months signals pregnancy. Blood discharged in the first three months is vicious (stagnant) blood, but incessant uterine bleeding is due to a tumor which should be discharged with *Gui zhi fu ling wan* (Cinnamon and Hoelen Formula)."

Hoelen Five Herb Formula

Wu ling san

Polyporus	*Polyporus*	*Zhu ling*	4.5
Hoelen	*Poria*	*Fu ling*	4.5
Alisma	*Alismatis Rhizoma*	*Ze xie*	6.0
Atractylodes (white)	*Atractylodis Rhizoma*	*Bai shu*	4.5
Cinnamon Twigs	*Cinnamomi Ramulus*	*Gui zhi*	3.0

Hoelen Five Formula is a harmonizing formula used for most water disorders in the body which cause overall water metabolism disturbances. The main symptoms are thirst, vomiting, dysuria, flushingup, palpitation, vertigo, anxiety, headache, abdominal pain, diarrhea, edema, and fever.

Functions:

Promotes yang, transforms qi, promotes diuresis, and dispels dampness.

Main Conformations:

Surface-fever and interior water conformation, edema, decreased urine, diarrhea, water stagnation in the stomach with palpitations beneath the umbilicus, softness in the abdominal wall, vomiting of water, extreme thirst, vertigo, and headaches.

Major Indications:

1. Pulse; floating and rapid, or sinking and soft.
2. Tongue; red with a thick coat.
3. Abdomen; soft and edematous (stagnant water) with water sounds in the stomach.
4. Water metabolism diseases.
5. Diarrhea and vomiting due to common cold.
6. Leukorrhea from cold/damp.
7. Diabetes.
8. Gastric disorders including seasickness.
9. Migraines and recurrent headaches.
10. Toxemia in pregnancy.
11. Overall bodyaches.

References from the Classics:

Shang Han Lun, page 13. "A little water will settle the stomach and cure patients with greater yang disease that manifests as dryness in the stomach after profuse perspiration induced by anxiety and irritability, and a desire to drink water. *Wu ling san* (Hoelen Five Herb Formula) is preferred for those cases with a floating pulse, dysuria, mild fever, and diabetic-like thirst."

Shang Han Lun, page 14. "*Wu ling san* (Hoelen Five Formula) is recommended for patients with a floating and rapid pulse, distress, and thirst after perspiring...*Wu ling san* (Hoelen Five Herb Formula) is given for *shang han* conditions with perspiration and thirst...*Wu ling san* (Hoelen Five Herb Formula) should be given for *chung feng* conditions exhibiting persistent, unrelieved fever over a period of six to seven days along with symptoms of anxiety, intense thirst, and vomiting after the ingestion of fluids."

Shang Han Lun, page 22. "Illness (fever, etc.) localized in the temporal area of the head should be treated with the sweating method using *Gui zhi ma huang ge ban tang* (Cinnamon and Ma-huang Combination). Water applied to the temples represses the heat so it cannot be dispersed. This results in severe anxiety, goose flesh, cutis anserina, and thirst which ceases immediately upon drinking. This condition calls for *Wan ke san* (Meretrix Formula); if a cure is not achieved, *Wu ling san* (Hoelen Five Herb Formula) is indicated. In cases with no heat conformation, but with cold inside which has accumulated in the chest, *San wu xiao bai san* (Platycodon and Croton Formula) is given."

Shang Han Lun, page 24. "Greater yang disease which has been treated by a physician first with the sweating method and then the purgation method, due to mistaken diagnosis of inside conformation, will exhibit relapsing fever and severe chills as a result of administering incorrect herbs, hardness beneath the heart with a sensation of tenderness on palpation, and a floating pulse. This condition should be treated with *Da huang huang lian xie xin tang* (Rhubarb, Coptis, and Scute Combination). Hardness beneath the heart, relapsing chills, and perspiration should be treated with *Da huang fu zi tang* (Rhubarb and Aconite Combination). For patients in whom the hardness is not relieved by *Ban xia xie xin tang* (Pinellia Combination), and who experience thirst, dryness of the mouth, anxiety, and dysuria *Wu ling san* (Hoelen Five Herb Formula) is indicated."

Shang Han Lun, page 57. "*Wu ling san* (Hoelen Five Herb Formula) is indicated for patients with vomiting, diarrhea, headache, fever, generalized aching, and thirst."

Shang Han Lun, page 88. "A thin individual who has palpitation beneath the navel, slobbering, and dizziness has a water problem and needs *Wu ling san* (Hoelen Five Herb Formula)."

Shang Han Lun, page 94. "*Wu ling san* (Hoelen Five Herb Formula) stimulates urination and perspiration in patients with a floating pulse, oliguria, slight fever, and polydipsia...*Wu ling san* (Hoelen Five Herb Formula) treats thirst in patients who vomit water immediately after drinking it. This condition is called water adversity."

Bupleurum and Gardenia Formula

Chai hu shu san

Bupleurum	*Bupleuri Radix*	*Chai hu*	4.0
Paeonia	*Paeoniae Radix*	*Shao yao*	4.0
Chih-shih	*Aurantii Fructus Immaturus*	*Zhi shi*	3.0
Licorice	*Glycyrrhizae Radix*	*Gan cao*	2.0
Cyperus	*Cyperi Rhizoma*	*Xiang fu zi*	3.0
Cnidium	*Cnidii Rhizoma (Ligustici Rhizoma)*	*Chuan xiong*	3.0
Blue citrus Peel	*Citri Immaturi Pericarpium*	*Qing pi*	12.0
Gardenia	*Gardeniae Fructus*	*Zhi zi*	3.0
Ginger	*Zingiberis Rhizoma*	*Sheng jiang*	1.0

This formula is indicated for intercostal neuralgia in patients with inflammation complicated by swelling and ulcers. It is very similar to *Si ni san* (Bupleurum and Chih-shih Formula), which is used for treating chest distention, abdominal spasm, cold hands and feet, and irritability caused by nervousness.

Major Indications

1. Pulse; tight and fast.
2. Tongue; red.
3. Abdomen; spasms.
4. Intercostal neuralgia.
5. Chest distress.
6. Swelling and ulcers.

Persica & Rhubarb Combination

Tao he cheng qi tang

Persica	*Persicae Semen*	*Tao ren*	5.0
Rhubarb	*Rhei Rhizoma*	*Da huang*	3.0
Cinnamon Twigs	*Cinnamomi Ramulus*	*Gui zhi*	4.0
Mirabilitum	*Natrium Sulfuricum*	*Mang xiao*	2.0
Licorice	*Glycyrrhizae Radix*	*Gan cao*	1.5

This formula is primarily used for treating stagnant blood in the lower jiao in strong constitution persons. Generally speaking, the disease will be long standing since it is on a blood level and will often manifest marked flushingup.

Functions:

Disperses stagnant blood and lumps in the abdomen.

Main Conformations:

Occluded blood, strong conformation, over excitability, hysteria, tinnitus and vertigo, dry mouth, flushingup with redness around the nose, general burning sensation, pulsation of the abdominal artery, sensation of distention in the lower abdomen, pain in the lower abdomen and lower back, constipation, spasm and cold in the legs and feet, and uterine bleeding.

Major Indications:

1. Pulse; deep and tight, or floating.
2. Tongue; red or purple with yellow coat.
3. Abdomen; distention, cramping, and pain in the lower jiao on palpation, palpitation of the abdominal artery.
4. Constipation.
5. Urogenital disorders due to stagnant blood.
6. Bleeding.
7. Hypertension.
8. Emotional instability.
9. Skin diseases due to heat in the blood.
10. Headache, vertigo, and tinnitus.

11. Low back pain.
12. Spasms and cold in the hands and feet.

References from the Classics:

Shang Han Lun, page 18. "An unrelieved greater yang disease, that exhibits a feverish lower jiao (the area between the stomach and bladder) will result in extravasated blood, which, in turn, will cause delirium in the patient. This condition may be helped by eliminating the extravasated blood from the bloody stool. However, if the surface symptoms do not improve with or without a bloody stool, purgative herbs should not further be administered. The surface symptoms should be relieved first, and, when this is done, the acute lower abdominal pain may be dispersed with *Tao he cheng qi tang* (Persica and Rhubarb Combination)."

Clematis and Stephania Combination

Shu jing huo xue tang

Tang-kuei	*Angelicae Radix*	*Dang gui*	2.0
Rehmannia	*Rehmanniae Radix*	*Di huang*	2.0
Atractylodes (white)	*Atractylodis Rhizoma*	*Bai shu*	2.0
Cnidium	*Cnidii Rhizoma (Ligustici Rhizoma)*	*Chuan xiong*	2.0
Persica	*Persicae Semen*	*Tao ren*	2.0
Hoelen	*Poria*	*Fu ling*	2.0
Peony	*Paeoniae Radix*	*Shao yao*	2.5
Achyranthes	*Achyranthis Radix*	*Niu xi*	1.5
Clematis	*Clematidis Radix*	*Wei ling xian*	1.5
Siler	*Ledebouriellae Radix*	*Fang feng*	1.5
Gentiana	*Gentianae Scabrae Radix*	*Long dan*	1.5
Ginger (fresh)	*Zingiberis Rhizoma*	*Sheng jiang*	1.5
Citrus	*Citri Leiocarpae Exocarpium*	*Chen pi*	1.5
Angelica	*Angelicae Dahuricae Radix*	*Bai zhi*	1.0
Licorice	*Glycyrrhizae Radix*	*Gan cao*	1.0
Stephania	*Aristolochiae Fangchi Radix*	*Fang ji*	1.5
Chiang-huo	*Notopterygii Rhizoma*	*Qiang huo*	1.5

This formula is used to warm and move stagnant blood due to excessive alcohol intake, sexual indulgence, internal or external injuries, or chronic blood deficiency. It increases blood circulation and causes stagnation to be dispersed. *Shu jing huo xue tang* (Clematis and Stephania Combination) treats pain in the muscles, joints and nerves, and especially pain below the waist.

Functions:

Clears meridians, activates blood, and dispels wind and dampness.

Main Conformations:

Pain in the muscles, joints and nerves; stagnated blood in the lower abdomen, spasms and chills in the legs, and water toxin.

Major Indications:

1. Pulse; slow, weak, and wiry, or possibly knotted.
2. Tongue; purple or pale.
3. Abdomen; tight with stagnation in the lower jiao.
4. Arthritis, and rheumatism.
5. Irregular menses due to stagnant blood.
6. Wind or cold type arthritis.
7. Sciatica lumbago, and numbness in the legs.
8. Postpartum pain.
9. Gout.

Ginseng and Ginger Combination

Li zhong wan

Ginseng	*Ginseng Radix*	*Ren shen*	3.0
Licorice	*Glycyrrhizae Radix*	*Gan cao*	3.0
Atractylodes (white)	*Atractylodes Rhizoma*	*Bai shu*	3.0
Ginger (dried)	*Zingiberis Siccatum Rhizoma*	*Gan jiang*	3.0

Li zhong wan (Ginseng and Ginger Combination) is used for weak water conformations. Treatment is directed to the middle jiao. As a hematinic and stomachic, it treats gastrointestinal weakness, pallor, polyuria, and tendencies toward fatigue and cold limbs, loose stools, frequent vomiting, headaches with fever, bodyaches, edema, insomnia, and bleeding.

Functions:

Warms spleen and stomach, dispels cold, tonifies qi, and strengthens spleen.

Main Conformations:

Weak chill conformation with greater yin disease, abnormal secretion of saliva and loss of appetite, general body pain, obstruction and pain in the chest, obstruction beneath the heart with fullness in the stomach, water stagnation in the stomach with sensation of chilling in the abdomen, edema, diarrhea, decreased urine, cold hands and feet, and heavy head.

Major Indications:

1. Pulse; slow and weak.
2. Tongue; moist and no coat.
3. Abdomen; weak, lax, cold, and painful; palpable water sounds in the stomach.
4. Acute and chronic gastrointestinal disorders.
5. Diabetes.
6. Diarrhea.
7. General pain and shoulder ache.
8. Water stagnation in the stomach.
9. Fatigue, anemia, and loss of appetite.
10. Bleeding from the uterus, intestines, and lungs, etc.

References from the Classics:

Shang Han Lun, page 57. "*Li zhong wan* (Ginseng and Ginger Combination) is preferred for vomiting, diarrhea, interior chills, and complete absence of thirst."

Shang Han Lun, page 60. "*Li zhong wan* (Ginseng and Ginger Combination) is recommended for patients with continued expectoration of thin sputum as a sequel to serious illness."

Chin Kuei Yao Lueh, page 61. "Thoracic paralysis accompanied by either obstructed qi beneath the heart, or by bound qi with distention in the chest and ribs, and flushing qi from the hypochondria to the heart should be treated with...*Li zhong wan* (Ginseng and Ginger Combination)."

Tang-kuei, Evodia and Ginger Combination

Dang gui si ni jia wu zhu yu sheng jiang tang

Tang-kuei	*Angelicae Radix*	*Dang gui*	3.0
Cinnamon Twigs	*Cinnamomi Ramulus*	*Gui zhi*	3.0
Peony	*Paeoniae Radix*	*Shao yao*	3.0
Asarum	*Asari Herba Cum Radice*	*Xi xin*	2.0
Licorice	*Glycyrrhizae Radix*	*Gan cao*	2.0
Akebia	*Akebiae Caulis*	*Mu tong*	3.0
Jujube	*Zizyphi Fructus*	*Da zao*	5.0
Evodia	*Evodiae Fructus*	*Wu zhu yu*	2.0
Ginger (fresh)	*Zingiberis Rhizoma*	*Sheng jiang*	4.0

This chill dispelling formula is used for treating patients with internal water poisoning who have chronic cold/blood stagnation on the jue yin energy level. Symptoms include chest distention, vomiting, ascites, diarrhea, and chills in the hands and feet.

Functions:

Warms the body and meridians, dispels cold, subdues ascending qi, and arrests vomiting.

Main Conformations:

Stagnant chills in the interior, cold sweats, annoying fullness in the chest, vomiting, abdominal spasm and pain, pain in the lower back, diarrhea, cold hands and feet (purple), and asthma with coughing up of sputum.

Major Indications:

1. Pulse; weak, thin, and small.
2. Tongue; thick white coat, flabby, and pale.
3. Abdomen; spasms, painful, weak, and cold.

4. Severe cold in the lower *jiao*.
5. Sciatica, cold joint and nerve disorders.
6. Cold limbs and chilblains.
7. Skin diseases.
8. Fatigue and anemia.

References from the Classics:

Shang Han Lun, page 54. "*Dang gui si ni jia wu zhu yu sheng jiang tang* (Tang-kuei and Jujube Combination) is recommended for patients with a sensation of chilled hands and feet (outside weakness of yang), and a small and weak pulse. This formula is given with *wu zhu yu* (evodia) and *sheng jiang* (fresh ginger) when the patient exhibits prolonged chills in the interior in addition to the outside chills."

Ginseng and Tang-kuei Ten Combination

Shi quan da bu tang

Ginseng	*Ginseng Radix*	*Ren shen*	3.0
Astragalus	*Astragali Radix*	*Huang qi*	3.0
Atractylodes (white)	*Atractylodis Rhizoma*	*Bai shu*	3.0
Peony	*Paeoniae Radix*	*Shao yao*	3.0
Hoelen	*Poria*	*Fu ling*	3.0
Rehmannia (cooked)	*Rehmanniae Radix*	*Shu di huang*	3.0
Tang-kuei	*Angelicae Radix*	*Dang gui*	3.0
Cnidium	*Cnidii Rhizoma (Ligustici Rhizoma)*	*Chuan xiong*	3.0
Cinnamon Twigs	*Cinnamomi Ramulus*	*Gui zhi*	3.0
Licorice	*Glycyrrhizae Radix*	*Gan cao*	1.0

This supplementing formula is used for very weak persons (men or women) with deficient spleen qi causing anemia, weak gastrointestinal tract, generalized fatigue, debility, weakness, and muscle spasms due to deficient qi. *Shi quan da bu tang* (Ginseng and Tang-kuei Ten) is used to treat the three types of ulcers caused by deficiency: 1) those with a small amount of pus; 2) those without pus; and 3) those with pus, but without tissue damage.

Functions:

Tonifies qi and blood and warms the body.

Main Conformations:

Dry skin, emaciation, generalized weakness, cardiac fatigue, weak gastrointestinal tract, abdominal weakness, loss of appetite, and anemia.

Major Indications:

1. Pulse; weak and deep.
2. Tongue; pale.
3. Abdomen; weak and flaccid.
4. Weakness due to loss of blood and anemia.
5. Weak gastrointestinal tract and hemorrhoidal bleeding.
6. Skin disease.
7. Menopausal symptoms.
8. Uterine carcinoma.
9. Postpartum/postsurgical fatigue.
10. Weakness in the knees.

Rehmannia Eight Formula

Ba wei di huang wan

Rehmannia (cooked)	*Rehmanniae Radix*	*Shu di huang*	5.0
Cinnamon twig	*Cinnamomi Ramulus*	*Gui zhi*	1.0
Aconite (processed)	*Aconiti Carmichaelii Praeparata Radix*	*Fu zi*	1.0
Hoelen	*Poria*	*Fu ling*	3.0
Dioscorea	*Dioscorea Batatis Rhizoma*	*Shan yao*	3.0
Alisma	*Alismatis Rhizoma*	*Ze xie*	3.0
Moutan	*Moutan Radicis Cortex*	*Mu dan pi*	3.0
Cornus	*Corni Fructus*	*Shan zhu yu*	3.0

This formula is used mainly for older people, but can be used for anyone experiencing deficient kidney energy. It is used more often in cases of deficient kidney yang rather than in those of deficient kidney yin. This formula actually reactivates the functions of degenerated kidneys, adrenals and reproductive organs, and is effective as a preventive and remedy for senility. It is given for the symptoms of severe fatigue and lassitude, sluggish gastrointestinal function, constipation, dysuria or polyuria, cold or warm limbs, thirst, lumbago, and weakness beneath the umbilicus.

Functions:

Warms and supplements kidney yang and nourishes yin and *jing*.

Main Conformation:

Extreme thirst, fatigue, normal digestion, lower back pain, defective and painful vision, impaired hearing, weakness and numbness below the umbilicus, infrequent or frequent urination, constipation, annoying fever in hands and feet, hands and feet which easily become cold in the winter, and spasms in the lower abdominis rectus muscle.

Major Indications:

1. Pulse; sinking and small, or tense, forceful and big.
2. Tongue; moist without fur.
3. Abdomen; weak.
4. Fatigue, sluggishness.
5. Lumbago, sciatica, and numbness of the legs.
6. Eye disease.
7. Urinary tract and kidney disorders.
8. Reproductive disorders, and menopause.
9. Diabetes.
10. Hyper- and hypotension.
11. Neurasthenia and impotence.
12. Eczema and itching.

References from the Classics:

Chin Kuei Yao Lueh, page 44. "A patient with weakness fatigue disease, lower back pain, lower abdominal cramping, and oliguria should primarily take *Ba wei di huang wan* (Rehmannia Eight Formula)."

Chin Kuei Yao Lueh, page 83. "Shortness of breath with mild water stagnancy has to be eliminated through urination. It requires *Ling gui shu gan tang* (Atractylodes and Hoelen Combination) or *ba wei di huang wan* (Rehmannia Eight Formula)."

Chin Kuei Yao Lueh, page 94. "Polydipsia and polyuria in a man who excretes an amount of urine equal to the volume of water drunk should be treated primarily with Ba wei di huang wan (Rehmannia Eight Formula)."

Chin Kuei Yao Lueh, page 157. "The disciples asked: 'Why would a woman with a normal appetite suffer from an annoying fever whereby she cannot lie down flat but must rest upright in order to breath?' The master said, 'The condition is known as "shift of the bladder," and it makes the patient incapable of urinating. Tangled ureters cause the problem, but it can be relieved by rendering urination with Ba wei di huang wan (Rehmannia Eight Formula).'"

Ma-huang, Aconite, and Asarum Combination

(AKA) Ma-huang and Asarum Combination

Ma huang fu zi xi xin tang

Aconite (processed)	*Aconiti Carmichaelii Praeparata Radix*	*Fu zi*	0.5-1.0
Asarum	*Asari Herba Cum Radice*	*Xi xin*	3.0
Ma-huang	*Ephedrae Herba*	*Ma huang*	4.0

This formula is used for treating overall exhaustion and achiness in very weak, debilitated or old persons. The formula is warming and should only be used in weak, cold, or deficient yang conformations. It is usually used in cases of acute onset of pathogenic wind/cold invasion.

Functions:

Restores yang and dispels chill.

Main Conformations:

Anemic facial complexion, mild fever, lassitude, chills in the back and head, general aching, edema in the legs, and cold arms and legs.

Major Indications:

1. Pulse; sinking, empty, and thin.
2. Tongue; pale and white coat.
3. Abdomen; water stagnancy.
4. Common cold in the elderly.
5. Wind/cold invasion, and upper respiratory disorders.
6. Headache due to wind and cold.
7. Anemia, and fatigue.
8. Edema.
9. Urinary disorders.

References from the Classics:

Shang Han Lun, page 47. "For patients contracting lesser yin disease with fever (a symptom of lesser yang disease), and a sinking pulse, *Ma huang fu zi xi xin tang* (Ma-huang, Aconite and Asarum Combination) is indicated."

Chapter 9

SKIN DISORDERS

The following formulas are arranged in order from the stronger and more aggressive to the more nutritive. The order is not meant as an absolute, but rather as a basic guide to how the formulas can be arranged for treatment.

During the tai yang (first) stage of skin disorders, the following should be considered:

- Cyperus and Perilla Formula
  (*Xiang su san*)

- Pueraria, Coptis and Scute Combination
  (*Ge gan huang lian huang qin tang*)

- Ma-huang and Coix Combination
  (*Ma huang yi gan tang*)

- Bupleurum and Schizonepeta Combination
  (*Shi wei bai du tang*)

- Siler and Platycodon Formula
  (*Fang feng tong sheng san*)

During the shao yang (second) stage of skin diseases, the following formulas should be considered:

- Sweet Combination
  (*Gan lu yin*)

- Bupleurum and Peony Formula
  (*Jia wei xiao yao san*)

- Cinnamon and Hoelen Formula
  (*Gui zhi fu ling wan*)

During the yang ming (third) stage of skin disorders, the following formulas should be considered:

- Rhubarb and Mirabilitum Combination
  (*Tiao wei cheng qi tang*)

- Forsythia and Laminaria Combination
  (*San zhong gui jian tang*)

- Forsythia and Lonicera Formula
  (*Zhi tou chuang yi fang*)

- Persica and Rhubarb Combination
  (*Tao he zheng qi tang*)

- Tang-kuei and Peony Formula
  (*Dang gui shao yao san*)

During the tai yin (fourth) stage of skin disorders, the following formulas should be considered:

- Gentiana Combination
  (*Long dan xie gan tang*)

- Tang-kuei and Gardenia Combination
  (*Wen jing yin*)

- Tang-kuei, Evodia, and Ginger Combination
  (*Dang gui si ni jia wu zhu yu sheng jiang tang*)

During the jue yin (sixth) stage of skin disorders, the following formulas should be considered:

- Lithospermum Ointment
  (*Zi yun gao*)
- Tang-kuei and Tribulus Combination
  (*Dang gui yin zi*)

Skin Disorder Symptoms

The following are basic disorders and indications commonly treated with the formulas in this section.

Acne

Symptoms: blocked pores on the face, chest, and back by sebum cutaneum and keratin. These substances harden, become yellow, and cause the skin to swell and suppurate.

Alopecia

Symptoms: partial or complete hair loss from the head.

Athlete's Foot (Hong Kong Foot)

Symptoms: blisters on the skin between the fingers and toes which soon dry, break open, and itch. When scratched, fluid flows out, and the area becomes moist.

Eczema

Symptoms: red swelling of the skin with the affected area becoming covered with pimples which turn into itching blisters. After a short time the blisters break, suppurate, and secrete a viscous fluid.

Facial Boils

Symptoms: boils containing a particle at the center of the pore which becomes red and begins to swell causing pain. As it enlarges, it begins to discharge pus. Severe cases are accompanied by fever, chills, and loss of appetite.

Herpes Zoster (Shingles)

Symptoms: burning pain that comes without warning and which is followed by skin lesions. Occasionally there will be neuralgia, fever, lassitude, and a loss of appetite followed by the skin reddening a few days after infection.

Hyperhidrosis

Symptoms: excessive perspiration which may occur in the armpits, on the face, palms of the hands and soles of the feet, or on the external genitalia.

Melanosis

Symptoms: melanomas or lentigines are oval, flat, brown, pigmented spots on the skin (mainly of the face). The main cause is the ultra violet rays of the sun.

Neurodermatitis

Symptoms: atopic dermatitis, exudative or thickened eruptions occurring on the face, neck, upper trunk, wrists, hands, and in the folds of the knees and elbows. Itching may be severe, long lasting, and lead to emotional disturbance.

Rosacea

Symptoms: bright and dark red coloration which spreads from the nose across the face. There is marked enlargement of the blood vessels, sebaceous glands, and connective tissue of the nose.

Scabies

Symptoms: small mites on the skin which secrete a viscous fluid and cause itching. The infected area itches intensely and becomes worse when it is warm at night.

Trichophytia Pompholyciformis (Ringworm)

Symptoms: small white vesicles on the palms and soles which turn purulent (pussy) in most cases. At times, the skin peels and cracks causing itching.

Urticaria

Symptoms: map-like erythema on the skin which is accompanied by severe itching. It subsides after several hours, and the patient recovers completely in one to seven days.

Formulas for Skin Disorders

Formula	Stage	Classification	Qi, Water Blood	Disorder	Patient Type
Cyperus and Perilla C.	tai yang	sudorific	qi	acute	medium
Pueraria, Coptis, and Scute C.	tai yang/ shao yang	dual dissolving	qi	acute	strong
Ma-huang and Coix C.	tai yang/ jue yin	sudorific	qi/ blood	chronic	weak
Bupleurum and Schizonepeta C.	tai yang/ shao yang	carbuncle dermatosis	blood	acute	medium
Siler and Platycodon C.	tai yang/ yang ming	dual dissolving	qi	chronic	weak
Sweet C.	shao yang/ tai yin	fire purging	qi/ blood	acute	medium
Bupleurum and Peony C.	shao yang/ jue yin	harmonizing	blood	acute	strong
Cinnamon and Hoelen C.	shao yang	blood	qi/ blood	chronic	weak
Rhubarb and Mirabilitum C.	yang ming	interior attacking	water blood	acute/ chronic	strong
Forsythia and Laminaria C.	yang ming	carbuncle/ dermatosis	blood	chronic	medium/ strong
Forsythia and Lonicera C.	yang ming	carbuncle/ dermatosis	blood	acute	weak/ strong
Persica and Rhubarb C.	yang ming	blood	blood	chronic	strong
Tang-kuei and Peony C.	yang ming	gynecological	blood	chronic	weak
Gentiana C.	tai yin	fire purging	blood	acute	strong
Tang-kuei and Gardenia C.	tai yin	blood	blood	chronic	weak
Tang-kuei, Evodia, and Ginger C.	tai yin	chill dispelling	water/ blood	chronic	weak
Tang-kuei and Tribulus C.	jue yin	moistening	blood	chronic	weak
Lithospermum Ointment	jue yin	carbuncles dermatosis	blood	acute/ chronic	medium

Cyperus and Perilla Formula

Xiang su san

Cyperus	*Cyperi Rhizoma*	*Xiang fu zi*	3.5
Perilla	*Perillae*	*Zi su*	1.5
Citrus Rind (dried)	*Citri Leiocarpae Exocarpium*	*Chen pi*	3.0
Licorice	*Glycyrrhizae Radix*	*Gan cao*	1.0
Ginger (fresh)	*Zingiberis Rhizoma*	*Sheng jiang*	1.0

Xiang su san (Cyperus and Perilla Formula) is a surface relieving formula which is used in the acute stages of tai yang and yang ming diseases. It can be used for any type of constitution and works when stagnant qi causes common colds, nausea, vomiting, headaches, vertigo, chest distention, etc. For skin diseases, it is appropriate to use *Xiang su san* (Cyperus and Perilla Formula) when someone has an allergic reaction which manifests hives or urticaria; for food poisoning caused by eating toxic fish, and other acute skin symptoms associated with toxic blood, rising yang, and rebellion.

Functions:

Relieves external conformations, regulates qi, and relieves qi and food stagnancy.

Main Conformations:

Heavy headedness, tinnitus, vertigo, nausea, acid regurgitation and vomiting, headache, stiff shoulders, obstructed and distended sensation in the epigastric region, below the heart and within the chest, and abdominal pain.

Major Indications:

1. Pulse; sinking and tight.
2. Tongue; thin white coat.
3. Abdomen; abdominal pain from emotional distress and fullness in the hypochondriac region.
4. Common cold and nasal congestion.
5. Gastrointestinal weakness.
6. Blood diseases.

7. Neurasthenia.
8. Eructation and vomiting.

Pueraria, Coptis and Scute Combination

Ge gen huang lian huang qin tang

Pueraria	*Purariae Radix*	*Ge gen*	6.0
Coptis	*Coptidis Rhizoma*	*Huang lian*	3.0
Scute	*Scutellariae Radix*	*Huang qin*	3.0
Licorice	*Glycyrrhizae Radix*	*Gan cao*	2.0

This formula is used in acute situations to purge heat. It is used for average-strong persons and to treat measles and other skin disorders associated with fever, thirst, diarrhea, and surface conformations.

Functions:

Relieves exterior evils and clears interior heat.

Main Conformations:

Fever with perspiration, mental instability, stiffness and spasm in the neck and back, asthma, palpitation in the heart, tenesmus, and diarrhea.

Major Indications:

1. Pulse; rapid and floating.
2. Tongue; red and thin yellow coat.
3. Abdomen; tight, tenesmus in lower abdomen, palpable obstructions and palpations in the hypochondriac region.
4. Asthma and gasping.
5. Measles.
6. Erysipelas.
7. Dysentery, diarrhea, and acute gastroenteritis.
8. Fever and thirst.
9. Mental instability.
10. Influenza and febrile diseases.
11. Hypertension.
12. Toothache.

Ma-huang and Coix Combination

Ma xing yi gan tang

Ma-huang	*Ephedrae Herba*	*Ma huang*	4.0
Apricot seed	*Armeniacae Semen*	*Xing ren*	3.0
Licorice	*Glycyrrhizae Radix*	*Gan cao*	2.0
Coix	*Coicis Semen*	*Yi yi ren*	10.0

Ma xing yi gan tang (Ma-huang and Coix Combination) is a cooling formula which helps to relieve water and blood trapped internally. It is best for acute symptoms causing generalized pain, rheumatism, and various skin disorders; in such cases, it is beneficial for qi level dermatological disorders, like eczema, and vesicular eruptions associated with fever.

Functions:

Promotes the circulation of lung qi and dispels moisture.

Main Conformations:

Cough and difficult breathing, fever, dry skin, muscle rheumatism, painful joints, edema, warts, and paralysis of the body.

Major Indications:

1. Pulse; rapid and possibly superficial.
2. Tongue; red tipped, or with red dots.
3. Abdomen; n/a.
4. Warts and vaginal warts.
5. Dry skin.
6. Herpes sores.
7. Calluses, corns, and warts.
8. Frostbite.
9. Eczema.
10. Dandruff.
11. Cough, difficult breathing, and asthma.
12. Muscle and/or joint pain.

References from the Classics:

Chin Kuei Yao Lueh, page 15-16. "Generalized aching and fever which aggravates in the evening, and which may accompany rheumatism. It occurs when one who is perspiring is caught in a draft, or when one becomes cold in the presence of chronic injury. Treatment calls for *Ma xing yi gan tang* (Ma-huang and Coix Combination)...There will be mild perspiring so the patient should stay out of the wind."

Bupleurum and Schizonepeta Combination

Shi wei bai du tang

Bupleurum	*Bupleuri Radix*	*Chai hu*	3.0
Ginger (fresh)	*Zingiberis Rhizoma*	*Sheng jiang*	1.0
Siler	*Ledebouriellae Radix*	*Fang feng*	2.0
Tu-huo	*Angelicae tuhuo Radix*	*Du huo*	2.0
Hoelen	*Poria*	*Fu ling*	2.0
Platycodon	*Platycodi Radix*	*Jie geng*	3.0
Schizonepeta	*Schizonepetae Herba*	*Jing jie*	1.0
Cnidium	*Cnidii Rhizoma (Ligustici Rhizoma)*	*Chuan xiong*	3.0
Licorice	*Glycyrrhizae Radix*	*Gan cao*	1.0
Cherry Bark	*Pruni Cortex*	*Ouhi*	3.0

This formula is especially effective for eczema, pimples, and urticaria. *Shi wei bai du tang* (Bupleurum and Schizonepeta Combination) has a positive effect on the autonomic nervous system and on glandular excretions, strengthen the liver, and improve resistance in allergic constitutions. It is specific for acute or chronic skin diseases due to heat in the liver. It is a fast acting formula, but can be taken for a long period of time. Persons taking this formula should have an average-strong constitution, but it is safe for children. When *yi yi ren* (coix) is added, the result is enhanced in the treatment of suppurative skin disease.

Functions:

Dispels wind and detoxifies.

Main Conformations:

Nervous temperament, fever, hypersensitive constitution, thoracocostal distress, acne, suppuration, carbuncles, and hives.

Major Indications:

1. Pulse; tight and fast.
2. Tongue; normal, but may be red.
3. Abdomen; medium strength.
4. Dermatitis.
5. Mastitis.
6. Carbuncles, furuncles, or boils.
7. Moist skin in diseased areas.
8. Allergic opthalmia.
9. Itching.

Siler and Platycodon Formula

Fang feng tong sheng san

Tang-kuei	*Angelicae Radix*	*Dang gui*	1.2
Peony	*Paeoniae Radix*	*Shao yao*	1.2
Gardenia	*Gardeniae Fructus*	*Zhi zi*	1.2
Cnidium	*Cnidii Rhizoma (Ligustici Rhizoma)*	*Chuan xiong*	1.2
Forsythia	*Forsythiae Fructus*	*Lian qiao*	1.2
Ginger (fresh)	*Zingiberis Rhizoma*	*Sheng jiang*	1.2
Schizonepeta	*Schizonepetae Herba*	*Jing jie*	1.2
Siler	*Ledebouriellae Radix*	*Fang feng*	1.2
Mentha	*Menthae Herba*	*Bo he*	1.2
Mirabilitum	*Natrium Sulfuricum*	*Mang xiao*	1.5
Ma-huang	*Ephedrae Herba*	*Ma huang*	1.2
Licorice	*Glycyrrhizae Radix*	*Gan cao*	2.0
Rhubarb	*Rhei Rhizoma*	*Da huang*	1.5
Atractylodes (white)	*Atractylodis Rhizoma*	*Bai shu*	2.0
Talc	*Talcum and Kaolinum*	*Hua shi*	3.0
Platycodon	*Platycodi Radix*	*Jie geng*	2.0
Scute	*Ledebouriellae Radix*	*Huang qin*	2.0
Gypsum	*Gypsum Fibrosum*	*Shi gao*	2.0

This is a harmonizing formula which works by cooling and purging qi, water and blood. It is used for those of strong constitution, and is good for strong full heat in both obese and normal weight persons (although it is specifically for the obese). This formula mainly affects kidney yin and liver yang disharmonies with symptoms of shoulder stiffness, numbness in the hands and feet, fatigue, headache, firm muscles, cardiac disorders, and habitual constipation. It is similar to *Da chai hu tang* (Major Bupleurum Combination), but treats a broader spectrum of disorders.

Functions:

Relieves exterior comformations and promotes sweating, purges interior heat and relieves constipation by dispelling the toxins of food, water and wind through the skin, excretory and digestive systems.

Main Conformations:

Obese constitution, facial reddening, yellowish white skin, constipation, and firmness and fullness in the abdomen centered at the umbilicus

Major Indications:

1. Pulse; tight, broad, strong, and sinking.
2. Tongue; red or purple raised papillae.
3. Abdomen; firm, full, and tight, especially at the umbilicus.
4. Scabies, eczema, acne, and alopecia.
5. Obesity.
6. Hypertension and arteriosclerosis.
7. Numb hands and feet.
8. Sciatica, 50 year old shoulder, and arthritis.
9. Asthma.
10. Diabetes.

Sweet Combination

Gan lu yin

Rehmannia (cooked)	*Rehmanniae Radix*	*Shu di huang*	2.5
Ophiopogon	*Ophiopogonis Tuber*	*Mai men dong*	2.5
Asparagus	*Asparagi Radix*	*Tian men dong*	2.5
Eriobotrya	*Eriobotryae Folium*	*Pi pa ye*	2.5
Chih-shih	*Aurantii Fructus Immaturus*	*Zhi shi*	2.5
Licorice	*Glycyrrhizae Radix*	*Gan cao*	2.5
Capillaris	*Artemisiae Capillaris Herba*	*Yin chen hao*	2.5
Dendrobium	*Dendrobii Caulis*	*Shi hu*	2.5
Scute	*Scutellariae Radix*	*Huang qin*	2.5

This formula is effective in dispelling heat, moisture and inflammation, and in purifying the blood. It is suitable for moist heat disorders of the skin, damp heat with stagnant blood in the digestive system, and symptoms such as suppuration and swelling with fever.

Functions:

Clears heat and dampness, cleanses blood, and reduces inflammation.

Main Conformations:

Reddening of the eyes, sores on the tongue, mouth or gums, swollen and bleeding gums, skin rash, general fever, swelling and pain in the throat, jaundice, and abdominal fullness with internal fever.

Major Indications:

1. Pulse; rapid and full.
2. Tongue; red with sores.
3. Abdomen; fullness.
4. Eczema and suppurative ulcers.
5. Stomatitis.
6. Gingivitis, pyorrhea, and toothache.
7. Scurvy.
8. Angina.
9. Conjunctivitis.
10. Jaundice.

Bupleurum and Peony Formula

Jia wei xiao yao san

Tang-kuei	*Angelicae Radix*	*Dang gui*	3.0
Peony	*Paeoniae Radix*	*Shao yao*	3.0
Gardenia	*Gardeniae Fructus*	*Zhi zi*	2.0
Atractylodes (white)	*Atractylodis Rhizoma*	*Bai shu*	3.0
Hoelen	*Poria*	*Fu ling*	3.0
Mentha	*Menthae Herba*	*Bo he*	1.0
Bupleurum	*Bupleuri Radix*	*Chai hu*	3.0
Moutan	*Moutan Radicis Cortex*	*Mu dan pi*	2.0
Ginger (dried)	*Zingiberis Siccatum Rhizoma*	*Gan jiang*	1.0
Licorice	*Glycyrrhizae Radix*	*Gan cao*	2.0

This is a harmonizing formula which is used in situations where liver is dominating spleen, or to nourish liver yin in average-strong persons. It acts on the blood level by moving stagnant blood in the lower jiao. It has a broad spectrum of uses including gynecological disorders, aching of the arms and legs, mental instability, flushingup, dizziness, thirst, and abdominal distention; all due to stagnant blood. The *Japanese Medical News* reported that this formula is the best remedy for cirrhosis, abdominal tenseness, thirst with persistent and bitter taste in the mouth, headache, turbid urine, and nosebleed.

Functions:

Soothes liver, removes liver qi stagnancy, tonifies spleen and blood, purges excess fire, and regulates menstruation.

Main Conformations:

Mild thoracocostal distress, afternoon flushingup sensation, vertigo, facial flushing, irritability, insomnia, feverish feeling that seems to move around, abnormal menstruation, and lassitude of the arms and legs.

Major Indications:

1. Pulse; wiry, and rapid.
2. Tongue; red, purple, and flabby.
3. Abdomen; tight and distended.

4. Mental disorders.
5. Premenstrual syndrome.
6. Menstrual irregularity.
7. Eczema and acne.
8. Infertility and menopausal symptoms.
9. Headaches, insomnia, and flushingup.
10. Leukorrhea.
11. Constipation.
12. Chronic and acute damp heat infections in the urogenital tract.

Cinnamon and Hoelen Formula

Gui zhi fu ling wan

Cinnamon Twigs	*Cinnamomi Ramulus*	*Gui zhi*	4.0
Hoelen	*Poria*	*Fu ling*	4.0
Persica	*Persicae Semen*	*Tao ren*	4.0
Peony	*Paeoniae Radix*	*Shao yao*	4.0
Moutan	*Moutan Radicis Cortex*	*Mu dan pi*	4.0

This is a blood-moving formula which improves circulation and disperses blood stagnation. It warms lower body chills and water accumulation, and rids internal heat from the upper body. It is used for persons of strong constitution and "kidney type" body. It can be used for acute flare-ups or chronic blood stagnation causing menstrual difficulty and/or menstrual irregularity. It is useful for skin diseases with stagnant blood.

Functions:

Dispels stagnant blood and lumps in the abdomen.

Main Conformations:

Blood stagnation in the face and lips, cardiac hyperfunction, spasms in the left rectus abdominis muscle, lumps in the lower abdomen, weak pain on pressure, lower abdominal and low back pain, melena (evacuation resembling tar), and menstrual irregularity.

Major Indications:

1. Pulse; deep, tense, and slow.

2. Tongue; red, purple, and flabby.
3. Abdomen; tight with lumps and spasms.
4. Flushingup, headaches, and vertigo.
5. Arthritis, rheumatism, and neuralgia.
6. Endometriosis.
7. Menopausal symptoms.
8. Dysmenorrhea and PMS.
9. Hypertension, hysteria, and nervousness.
10. Eczema, dermatitis, pimples, and black spots.
11. Lumbago and shoulder pain.

References from the Classics:

Chin Kuei Yao Lueh, page 141. "Movement above the navel and sudden incessant uterine bleeding three months after the cessation of menses indicates the presence of a tumor. However, movement in the sixth month with regular menses in the first three months signals pregnancy. Blood discharged in the first three months is vicious (stagnant) blood, but incessant uterine bleeding is due to a tumor which should be discharged with *Gui zhi fu ling wan* (Cinnamon and Hoelen Formula)."

Rhubarb and Mirabilitum Combination

Tiao wei cheng qi tang

Rhubarb	*Rhei Rhizoma*	*Da huang*	2.5
Mirabilitum	*Natrium Sulfuricum*	*Mang xiao*	1.0
Licorice	*Glycyrrhizae Radix*	*Gan cao*	1.0

Although this is a cool yang ming formula, it is used for weak-average constitutions. It purges stagnant blood and water, and works to relieve surface toxins. It is used primarily in skin diseases involving fever and constipation, especially in the aged or weak, and purges internal toxins in a relatively gentle fashion by lubricating yin deficiency.

Functions:

Purges heat and induces bowel movements.

Main Conformations:

Constipation or diarrhea, mild abdominal pain and distention, upset stomach, fever, spontaneous sweating, delirium, and dry mouth and tongue.

Major Indications:

1. Pulse; deep and firm, or possibly choppy or ropy.
2. Tongue; dry, thick coat, and possibly red bumps in the rear.
3. Abdomen; tense, distended, and painful on palpation.
4. Constipation or diarrhea.
5. Food poisoning, and food stagnation.
6. Febrile diseases with constipation.
7. Mild asthma.
8. Constipation in the elderly.
9. Acute gastroenteritis.

References from the Classics:

Shang Han Lun, page 9. "A small portion of *Tiao wei cheng qi tang* (Rhubarb and Mirabilitum Combination) is given to patients with stomach disorders and delirium."

Shang Han Lun, page 13. "The patient who has severe chills after perspiring is of the weak type; (patients) with fever but no severe chills (following perspiring) are of the strong type. The stomach reaction of the strong type should be harmonized by administering *Tiao wei cheng qi tang* (Rhubarb and Mirabilitum Combination)."

Shang Han Lun, page 19. "Greater yang disease which persists for more than ten days with heart distress, gagging, aching in the chest, loose stools (the condition has now entered into the sunlight yang category), mild abdominal distention, depression, and mild anxiety; and prior to these symptoms, severe vomiting and diarrhea (occurring spontaneously) should be treated with *Tiao wei cheng qi tang* (Rhubarb and Mirabilitum Combination)."

Shang Han Lun, pages 40-41. "Patients with greater yang disease lasting for more than three days who have had incomplete relief following treatment with the sweating method, and who have a persisting fever due to stomach trouble, should be given *Tiao wei cheng qi tang* (Rhubarb and Mirabilitum Combination)."

Shang Han Lun, page 59. "A mild purgation agent with *Tiao wei cheng qi tang* (Rhubarb and Mirabilitum Combination) is given to patients with a sinking solid pulse (inside firmness), or post-illness conditions."

Forsythia and Laminaria Combination

San zhong kui jian tang

Tang-kuei	*Angelicae Radix*	*Dang gui*	1.5
Peony	*Paeoniae Radix*	*Shao yao*	1.5
Bupleurum	*Bupleuri Radix*	*Chai hu*	1.5
Scute	*Scutellariae Radix*	*Huang qin*	1.5
Coptis	*Coptidis Rhizoma*	*Huang lian*	1.5
Forsythia	*Forsythiae Fructus*	*Lian qiao*	1.5
Phellodendron	*Phellodendri Cortex*	*Huang bo*	1.5
Platycodon	*Platycodi Radix*	*Jie geng*	1.5
Gentiana	*Gentianae Scabrae Radix*	*Long dan*	1.5
Anemarrhena	*Anemarrhenae Rhizoma*	*Zhi mu*	1.5
Pueraria	*Purariae Radix*	*Ge gen*	1.5
Scirpus	*Sparganii Rhizoma*	*San ling*	1.5
Zedoaria	*Zedoariae Rhizoma*	*E shu*	1.5
Laminaria	*Laminariae Thallus*	*Hai dai*	1.5
Seaweed	*Sargassum*	*Hai zao*	1.5
Cimicifuga	*Cimicifugae Rhizoma*	*Sheng ma*	1.5
Ginger (fresh)	*Zingiberis Rhizoma*	*Sheng jiang*	1.5
Licorice	*Glycyrrhizae Radix*	*Gan cao*	1.5
Trichosanthes Root	*Trichosanthis Radix*	*Gua lou gen*	1.5

This formula is used for the treatment of swollen lymph glands, goiter, carbuncles, acute inflammation, and suppurative ulcers. It is especially effective for lymphadenectasis involving the supraauricular and suprasecapular areas.

Functions:

Dispels hardness and reduces swelling.

Main Conformations:

Cervical lymphadnectasis (involving the subauricular and suprascapular areas), reddish and brown skin, and obstruction and distention beneath the heart

Major Indications:

1. Pulse; floating, tight, and fast.
2. Tongue; red with white coat.
3. Abdomen; obstruction and distention beneath the heart.
4. Carbuncles and lymphadenitis in the neck.

Forsythia and Lonicera Formula

Zhi tou chuang yi fang

Forsythia	*Forsythiae Fructus*	*Lian qiao*	2.0
Siler	*Ledebouriellae Radix*	*Fang feng*	2.0
Carthamus	*Carthami Flos*	*Hong hua*	1.0
Cnidium	*Cnidii Rhizoma (Ligustici Rhizoma)*	*Chuan xiong*	3.0
Lonicera	*Lonicerae Flos*	*Jin yin hua*	2.0
Licorice	*Glycyrrhizae Radix*	*Gan cao*	1.0
Atractylodes (red)	*Atractylodis Lanceae Rhizoma*	*Cang zhu*	3.0
Schizonepeta	*Schizonepetae Herba*	*Jing jie*	1.0
Rhubarb	*Rhei Rhizoma*	*Da huang*	0.5

This formula has been widely used in Japan as a cure for head sores. It is believed that head sores develop as a result of embryonic toxemia, and are possibly related to genetic factors which determine individual hypersensitivity. Skin disease that affect the head, neck, armpits, and genitalia as well as other parts of the body can be treated with this formula. The effected part first has red papules followed by blisters, which eventually ulcerate and form into scabs. If there is a discharge, the herb *da huang* (rhubarb) should be excluded. For the above condition it is recommended that this formula be taken continuously for one or two months.

Functions:

Harmonizes and detoxifies.

Main Conformations:

Strong conformation, head sores with secretion of pus and scabbing, reddening of pimples or erosion, or scabs on the face, neck, armpits and external genital organs, and especially in females.

Major Indications:

1. Pulse; floating and full.
2. Tongue; red and yellow coat.
3. Abdomen; firm and tense.
4. Head sores with secretion of pus and scabbing.
5. Eczema on the head of children.
6. Inflammatory dermatitis.
7. Genital warts and pimples.
8. Constipation.

Persica & Rhubarb Combination

Tao he cheng qi tang

Persica	*Persicae Semen*	*Tao ren*	5.0
Rhubarb	*Rhei Rhizoma*	*Da huang*	3.0
Cinnamon Twig	*Cinnamomi Ramulus*	*Gui zhi*	4.0
Mirabilitum	*Natrium Sulfuricum*	*Mang xiao*	2.0
Licorice	*Glycyrrhizae Radix*	*Gan cao*	1.5

This is a heat purging formula which relieves stagnant blood in the lower jiao with heat rising up to the blood level; this causes flushingup and habitual constipation. The person taking this formula must be of a strong constitution. It acts on a superficial level treating toxins in the large intestine as well as heat in the liver. Because this formula works on a blood level, it is used to treat disorders long standing in nature. It also disperses stagnant blood and lumps in the abdomen.

Main Conformations:

Occluded blood, strong conformation, over excitability, hysteria, tinnitus and vertigo, dry mouth, flushingup with redness around the nose, general burning sensation, pulsation of the abdominal artery, sensation of distention in the lower abdomen, pain in the lower abdomen and lower back, constipation, spasms and cold legs and feet, and uterine bleeding.

Major Indications:

1. Pulse; deep and tight, or floating and full.
2. Tongue; red or purple with yellow coat, and possibly dry.
3. Abdomen; tight, distended, cramping, and with pain in the lower jiao.
4. Dermatitis, eczema, urticaria, and acne.
5. Athlete's foot, ringworm, and warts.
6. Infections of the urinary tract and prostate.
7. Menstrual irregularities, dysmenorrhea, and endometriosis.
8. Menopausal symptoms.
9. Abnormal bleeding in the body.
10. Eye disorders.

References from the Classics:

Shang Han Lun, page 18. "An unrelieved greater yang disease that exhibits a feverish lower jiao (the area between the stomach and the bladder) will result in extravasated blood, which, in turn, will cause delirium in the patient. This condition may be helped by eliminating the extravasated blood in bloody stools. However, if the surface symptoms do not improve with or without a bloody stool, purgative herbs should no further be administered. The surface symptoms should be relieved first, and when this is done the acute lower abdominal pain may be dispersed with *Tao he cheng qi tang* (Persica and Rhubarb Combination)."

Tang-kuei and Peony Formula

Dang gui shao yao san

Tang-kuei	*Angelicae Radix*	*Dang gui*	3.0
Peony	*Paeoniae Radix*	*Shao yao*	4.0
Hoelen	*Poria*	*Fu ling*	4.0
Atractylodes (white)	*Atractylodis Rhizoma*	*Bai shu*	4.0
Cnidium	*Cnidii Rhizoma (Ligustici Rhizoma)*	*Chuan xiong*	3.0
Alisma	*Alismatis Rhizoma*	*Ze xie*	4.0

This formula is used to move and warm blood in average to weak persons; it is used mainly for women with blood stagnation due to weakness. *Dang gui shao yao san* (Tang-kuei and Peony Combination) also addresses excess water affecting the stomach and/or kidney energy. It is very effective in the treatment of skin diseases due to yin weakness, postpartum weakness, general lassitude, menstrual disorders, OB-GYN related urinary tract problems, and infertility. It is a specific in aiding women to carry a fetus full term, particularly if they have had a miscarriage in the past.

Functions:

Tonifies blood and qi, activates blood, and assists water metabolism.

Main Conformations:

Yin weakness conformation, chill conformation, irregular menstruation, prolonged menstrual flow, abnormal leukorrhea, lower abdominal and low back pain, rectus abdominis muscle spasms with softness of the abdominal wall, tinnitus, vertigo, heavy head, and anemia.

Major Indications:

1. Pulse; sinking, weak, and thready.
2. Tongue; pale, swollen, scalloped,and thin coat.
3. Abdomen; soft, painful with spasms of the rectus abdominis muscles, and splashing sounds beneath the heart.
4. Body type; thin and soft muscles.
5. Leukorrhea.

6. Prolonged menstrual flow and irregular menses.
7. Anemia, fatigue, and pale and/or dry skin.
8. Edema, nephritis, and cystitis.
9. Increased or decreased urination.
10. Chills due to poor circulation.
11. Infertility and habitual abortion.
12. Postpartum weakness.
13. Tinnitus, vertigo

References from the Classics:

Chin Kuei Yao Lueh, page 142. "*Dang gui shao yao san* (Tang-kuei and Peony Formula) helps pregnant women with abdominal cramping pain."

Chin Keui Yao Lueh, page 157. "*Dang gui shao yao san* (Tang-kuei and Peony Formula) treats various women's abdominal problems."

Gentiana Combination

Long dan xie gan tang

Gentiana	*Gentianae Scabrae Radix*	*Long dan*	1.0
Alisma	*Alismatis Rhizoma*	*Ze xie*	3.0
Akebia	*Akebiae Caulis*	*Mu tong*	5.0
Plantago	*Plantaginis Semen*	*Che qian zi*	3.0
Tang-kuei	*Angelicae Radix*	*Dang gui*	5.0
Rehmannia (raw)	*Rehmanniae Radix*	*Sheng di huang*	5.0
Gardenia	*Gardeniae Fructus*	*Zhi zi*	1.0
Scute	*Scutellariae Radix*	*Huang qin*	3.0
Licorice	*Glycyrrhizae Radix*	*Gan cao*	1.0

This is a fire purging formula which is used for persons of strong to average constitution; it is contraindicated in persons with a delicate constitution. The formula eliminates heat and inflammation and should be administered only briefly. It is good for acute flare-ups of true heat signs, symptoms of liver yang rising, heat in the blood, or damp/heat in the lower jiao. Symptoms include pain in the armpits, deafness, swollen ears, blood in the urine, and redness of the mouth and eyes.

Functions:

Clears liver heat and dampness.

Main Conformations:

Strong conformation, pale dark skin, tension and hypersensitivity on the outside of the abdominal rectus muscle, pain and swelling in the lower abdomen, and dampness on the inside of the hands and feet.

Major Indications:

1. Pulse; tense, rapid, and forceful and rolling.
2. Tongue; red with thick yellow coat.
3. Abdomen; tension, pain and swelling in lower abdomen.
4. Acute leukorrhea.
5. Gonorrhea, endometritis, and venereal ulcers.
6. Hematuria, cystitis, and urethritis.
7. Herpes.
8. Itching, inflammation, and pain in genital area.
9. Eczema and orchitis.
10. Groin lymphadenitis.

Tang-kuei and Gardenia Combination

Wen qing yin

Tang-kuei	*Angelicae Radix*	*Dang gui*	4.0
Rehmannia	*Rehmanniae Radix*	*Di huang*	4.0
Peony	*Paeoniae Radix*	*Shao yao*	3.0
Cnidium	*Cnidii Rhizoma (Ligustici Rhizoma)*	*Chuan xiong*	3.0
Coptis	*Coptidis Rhizoma*	*Huang lian*	1.5
Scute	*Scutellariae Radix*	*Huang qin*	3.0
Phellodendron	*Phellodendri Cortex*	*Huang bo*	1.5
Gardenia	*Gardeniae Fructus*	*Zhi zi*	2.0

Wen qing yin (Tang-kuei and Gardenia Combination) cools, moves, and builds blood. It is for weak-average type persons with chronic blood stagnation and damp heat. This formula is a combination of *Si wu tang*

(Tang-kuei Four Combination) and *Huang lian jie du tang* (Coptis and Scute Combination). The main sign indicating this formula are areas of dark brown skin. Bleeding skin, emotional disorders with internal heat, and liver blood deficiency symptoms can be treated with this formula as well.

Functions:

Clears heat, cools blood, activates blood, and dispels stagnant blood.

Main conformations:

Uterine bleeding, ulcers on the external genitals, dry itching skin, blackish, brown-yellow or brown skin, ulcers of the mouth, tongue, and cheeks, neurotic excitability, and tension beneath the hypochondrium and rectus abdominis muscle.

Major Indications:

1. Pulse; rapid, tight or slippery.
2. Tongue; red, especially on the sides, yellow coat, and possibly red tipped.
3. Abdomen; tense, especially beneath the hypochondriac region on the rectus abdominis muscle.
4. Dry skin, itching, and eczema.
5. Uterine bleeding.
6. Hypertension.
7. Emotional instability.
8. Leukorrhea.
9. Generalized skin diseases due to toxic heat (eg. dermatitis, and urticaria).
10. Ulceration of the mouth, tongue, cheeks, and external genitals.
11. Liver disorders.
12. Peptic and duodenal ulcers.

Tang-kuei, Evodia, and Ginger Combination

Dang gui si ni jia wu zhu yu sheng jiang tang

Tang-kuei	*Angelicae Radix*	*Dang gui*	3.0
Cinnamon Twigs	*Cinnamomi Ramulus*	*Gui zhi*	3.0
Peony	*Paeoniae Radix*	*Shao yao*	3.0
Asarum	*Asari Herba Cum Radice*	*Xi xin*	2.0
Licorice	*Glycyrrhizae Radix*	*Gan cao*	2.0
Akebia	*Akebiae Caulis*	*Mu tong*	3.0
Jujube	*Zizyphi Fructus*	*Da zao*	5.0
Evodia	*Evodiae Fructus*	*Wu zhu yu*	2.0
Ginger (fresh)	*Zingiberis Rhizoma*	*Sheng jiang*	4.0

This is a chill dispelling formula which is used to treat chronic cold blood stagnation in the middle and lower jiaos. Symptoms include chills in the extremities due to febrile disease, excess sweating, and gynecological and skin disorders where there is internal and external coldness and internal water poisoning. The formula warms the blood and improves overall blood circulation in weak persons. The body type of this individual is heavyset.

Functions:

Warms the body and meridians, dispels cold, subdues ascending qi, and arrests vomiting.

Main Conformations:

Stagnant chills in the interior, cold sweats, annoying fullness in the chest, vomiting, abdominal spasms and pain, pain in lower back, diarrhea, cold hands and feet (purple), asthma, and coughing up sputum.

Major Indications:

1. Pulse; thin, weak, and deep.
2. Tongue; flabby and pale.
3. Abdomen; pain and spasms.
4. Uterine bleeding and pain.
5. Dysmenorrhea.

6. Cold limbs and cold sweats.
7. Low back pain, sciatica, and cold nerve and joint disorders.
8. Diarrhea.
9. Calluses and corns.
10. Red dots on the skin (petechia) and skin disorders.
11. Fatigue and anemia.

References from the Classics:

Shang Han Lun, page 54. "*Dang gui si ni tang* (Tang-kuei and Jujube Combination) is recommended for patients with a sensation of chilled hands and feet (an outside weakness of yang), and a small and weak pulse. This formula is given with *wu chu yu* (evodia) and *sheng jiang* (fresh ginger) when the patient exhibits prolonged chills on the inside in addition to the outside chills."

Tang-kuei and Tribulus Combination

Dang gui yin zi

Tang-kuei	*Angelicae Radix*	*Dang gui*	5.0
Peony	*Paeoniae Radix*	*Shao yao*	3.0
Cnidium	*Cnidii Rhizoma (Ligustici Rhizoma)*	*Chuan xiong*	3.0
Tribulus	*Tribuli Fructus*	*Ji li*	3.0
Siler	*Ledebouriellae Radix*	*Fang feng*	3.0
Rehmannia	*Rehmanniae Radix*	*Di huang*	4.0
Ho-shou-wu	*Polygoni Multiflori Radix*	*He shou wu*	2.0
Schizonepeta	*Schizonepetae Herba*	*Jing jie*	1.5
Astragalus	*Astragali Radix*	*Huang qi*	1.5
Licorice	*Glycyrrhizae Radix*	*Gan cao*	1.0

This formula is effective for the treatment of dry skin and itching due to deficient blood, blood dryness, or wind/heat. It can be used for patients with skin disorders who have a delicate constitution, and it is a safe formula that can be taken for a long period of time.

Functions:

Tonifies blood, moistens blood dryness, dispels wind and relieves itching.

Main Conformations:

Weak conformation, dry skin, itching, and anemia.

Major Indications:

1. Pulse; thready and weak.
2. Tongue; pale and flabby.
3. Itching.
4. Anemia.
5. Dry skin and insufficient skin secretions.
6. Chronic eczema.
7. Carbuncles.

Lithospermum Ointment

Zi yun gao

Sesame Oil	*Oleum Sesami*	*Hu ma you*	1000
Tang-kuei	*Angelicae Radix*	*Dang gui*	100
Lard		*Zhu you*	25
Flava Wax	*Cera Flava*	*Huang la*	380
Lithospermum	*Lithospermi Radix*	*Zi cao*	100

Zi yun gao (Lithospermum Ointment) is reportedly the most important ointment for external use. It is effective for a wide variety of skin diseases, and can be taken in conjunction with other skin formulas.

Functions:

Reduces inflammation, prevents bleeding, eliminates bacteria, relieves pain, and promotes tissue regeneration.

Major Indications:

1. Dry skin and eczema.
2. Wrinkles.
3. Ulcerations.

4. Skin cancer.
5. Fungus.
6. Burns.
7. Acne.
8. Calluses and corns.
9. Prickly heat.
10. Body heat and alopecia.

Chapter 10

GYNECOLOGICAL DISORDERS

The following formulas are arranged in order from the stronger and more aggressive to the more nutritive. The order is not meant as an absolute, but rather as a basic guide to how the formulas can be arranged for treatment.

During the tai yang (first) stage of gynecological disorders, the following should be considered:

- Coptis and Scute Combination
  (*Huang lian jie du tang*)

- Bupleurum and Cinnamon Combination
  (*Chai hu gui zhi tang*)

During the shao yang (second) stage of gynecological disorders, the following should be considered:

- Bupleurum and Dragon Bone Combination
  (*Chai hu jia long gu mu li tang*)

- Bupleurum and Hoelen Combination
  (*Chai ling tang*)

- Cinnamon and Hoelen Formula
  (*Gui zhi fu ling wan*)

- Bupleurum and Peony Formula
  (*Jia wei xiao yao san*)

During the yang ming (third) stage of gynecological disorders, the following should be considered:

- Gentiana Combination
  (*Long dan xie gan tang*)

- Rhubarb and Leech Combination
  (*Di dang tang*)

- Persica and Rhubarb Combination
  (*Tao he cheng qi tang*)

- Lithospermum and Oyster Shell Combination
  (*Zi gen mu li tang*)

During the tai yin (fourth) stage of gynecological disorders, the following should be considered:

- Lotus Seed Combination
  (*Qing xin lian zi yin*)

- Licorice and Jujube Combination
  (*Gan mai da zao tang*)

- Ginseng and Longan Combination
  (*Gui pi tang*)

Gynecological Disorder Symptoms

The following are basic disorders and indications commonly treated with the formulas in this section.

Breast Cancer

Symptoms: hard, painless lump in the breast, and sometimes the nipple will bleed or become ulcerated. Breast cancer is usually located in the upper outer quadrant of the breast.

Climacteric Disorder (Menopause)

Symptoms: chilling, fever, hot flashes, headache, aching shoulders, sweating, palpitations, painful menstruation, irritability, depression, and insomnia.

Endometritis

Symptoms: discomfort or pain in the lower abdomen, and malodorous leukorrhea which consists of a mixture of pus and mucus, and which is milky or yellow in color. There is also itching on the outside of the vagina, painful menstruation, bleeding during intercourse, vaginal infection, chilling, fever, irritability, and loss of appetite.

Leukorrhea

Symptoms: milky or yellow vaginal discharge with pus or blood. If caused by cancer or abortion, it will have an abnormal odor.

Mastitis

Symptoms: parts of the breast become hard, swollen, and painful. The inflamed area is feverish and red. In severe cases there is pus, general tiredness, loss of appetite, and headache.

Ovaritis and Oviduct Inflammation

Symptoms: severe pain and fever in the lower abdomen, occasional pus, and continuous fever. In the chronic state there will be ovarian swelling and pressing pain, continuous pain in the lower abdomen, lumbago, and pain on excretion and during intercourse.

Uterine Carcinoma

Symptoms: leukorrhea that is malodorous, mixed with blood or pus which causes itching at the vagina, and vaginal bleeding after intercourse. When the malignancy has become advanced there will be pain in the lower abdomen.

Formulas for Gynecological Disorders

Formula	Stage	Classification	Qi, Water Blood	Disorder	Patient Type
Coptis and Scute C.	tai yang/ shao yang	fire purging	qi	acute	strong
Bupleurum and Cinnamon C.	tai yang/ shao yang	dual dissolving	qi	acute/ chronic	medium/ weak
Bupleurum and Dragon bone C.	shao yang	sedative	qi	chronic	weak
Bupleurum and Hoelen C.	shao yang	diuretic	water	chronic	weak
Cinnamon and Hoelen C.	shao yang	blood	qi/ blood	chronic	weak
Bupleurum and Peony C.	shao yang/ jue yin	harmonizing	blood	acute	strong
Gentiana C.	yang ming	fire/ purging	blood	acute	strong
Rhubarb and Leech C.	yang ming	blood	blood	acute/ chronic	strong
Persica and Rhubarb C.	yang ming	blood	blood	chronic	strong
Lithospermum and Oyster Shell C.	yang ming/ jue yin	carbuncle dermatosis	blood	chronic	weak
Lotus Seed C.	tai yin	fire purging	water	acute	weak
Licorice and Jujube C.	shao yin	sedative	qi	chronic	weak
Ginseng and Longan C.	shao yin	blood	blood	chronic	weak

Coptis and Scute Combination

Huang lian jie du tang

Scute	*Scutellariae Radix*	*Huang qin*	3.0
Coptis	*Coptidis Rhizoma*	*Huang lian*	1.5
Gardenia	*Gardeniae Fructus*	*Zhi zi*	2.0
Phellodendron	*Phellodendri Cortex*	*Huang bo*	1.5

This is a heat clearing formula which is used to treat strong persons with true heat signs causing inflammation, anxiety, bleeding, and overall congestion. It can address heat in any organ system, but is mainly used in liver fire situations; it brings down heat, moves blood, and detoxifies. Generally used only in acute situations, such as hemorrhage, it also works on interior heat infections.

Functions:

Clears heat, purges fire, arrests bleeding and relieves irritability.

Main Conformations:

Yang strong conformation, cardiac hyperfunction, restlessness, insomnia, spitting and vomiting blood, facial reddening, chest discomfort with sensation of resistance beneath the heart, forceful abdomen, melena (stools resembling tar in appearance), and red urine.

Major Indications:

1. Pulse; forceful, deep, and possibly rapid.
2. Tongue; red and possible yellow coat.
3. Abdomen; strong and tight.
4. Hypertension, anxiety.
5. Constipation.
6. Bleeding disorders (due to true heat).
7. Insomnia.
8. Resistance beneath the heart and palpitations.
9. Cerebral hemorrhage.
10. Herpes and urticaria.
11. Joint and nerve disorders.
12. Acute PID and post D&C infection and inflammation.

Bupleurum and Cinnamon Combination

Chai hu gui zhi tang

Bupleurum	*Bupleuri Radix*	*Chai hu*	5.0
Pinellia	*Pinellia Tuber*	*Ban xia*	4.0
Licorice	*Glycyrrhizae Radix*	*Gan cao*	1.5
Jujube	*Zizyphi Fructus*	*Da zao*	2.0
Cinnamon Twigs	*Cinnamomi Ramulus*	*Gui zhi*	2.5
Scute	*Scutellariae Radix*	*Huang qin*	2.0
Ginseng	*Ginseng Radix*	*Ren shen*	2.0
Peony	*Paeoniae Radix*	*Shao yao*	2.5
Ginger (dried)	*Zingiberis Siccatum Rhizoma*	*Gan jiang*	1.0

This formula is good for people with somewhat delicate constitutions who are experiencing extreme fatigue, gastrointestinal weakness, headache, heaviness in the head, neuralgia, fever and chills, distention beneath the heart, and lower abdominal pain. *Chai hu gui zhi tang* (Bupleurum and Cinnamon Combination) is a mixture of *Xiao chai hu tang* (Minor Bupleurum Combination), and *Gui zhi tang* (Cinnamon Combination). The patient in question will often have a liver body type (thin and wiry), be blood deficient, and susceptible to external cold. A common syndrome seen where this formula would be effective is liver (wood) overacting on earth; this shows both liver and spleen/stomach symptoms in persons affected.

Functions:

Dispels wind, relieves exterior evil, harmonizes nutritive and protective qi, and harmonizes exterior and interior.

Main Conformations:

Greater yang and lesser yang conformation, neurotic behavior, mild vomiting, mild chills, pain in the joints, acute pain in the heart and abdomen, mild thoracocostal distress, and heavy head with headaches.

Major Indications:

1. Pulse; floating and weak.
2. Tongue; red, quivering, or pale with scallops.

3. Abdomen; tense or flaccid and distended.
4. Mental instability and nervous exhaustion.
5. Severe stomach/abdominal pain and gastrointestinal disorders.
6. Prolonged common cold with nausea and respiratory disorders.
7. Anorexia.
8. Premenstrual syndrome (PMS) symptoms.
9. Intercostal neuralgia, and arthralgia.

References from the Classics:

Shang Han Lun, page 22. "*Shang han* lasting six to seven days with fever, mild chills, persisting aching in the limbs, mild vomiting, and distention beneath the heart requires *Chai hu gui zhi tang* (Bupleurum and Cinnamon Combination)."

Chin Kuei Yao Lueh, page 71. "*Chai hu gui zhi tang* (Bupleurum and Cinnamon Combination) treats acute pain in the heart and the abdomen."

Bupleurum and Dragon Bone Combination

Chai hu jia long gu mu li tang

Bupleurum	*Bupleuri Radix*	*Chai hu*	5.0
Hoelen	*Poria*	*Fu ling*	3.0
Pinellia	*Pinellia Tuber*	*Ban xia*	4.0
Rhubarb	*Rhei Rhizoma*	*Da huang*	1.0
Cinnamon Twigs	*Cinnamomi Ramulus*	*Gui zhi*	3.0
Scute	*Scutellariae Radix*	*Huang qin*	2.5
Jujube	*Zizyphi Fructus*	*Da zao*	2.5
Ginseng	*Ginseng Radix*	*Ren shen*	2.5
Ginger (fresh)	*Zingiberis Rhizoma*	*Sheng jiang*	2.5
Oyster Shell	*Ostreae Testa*	*Mu li*	2.5
Dragon Bone	*Draconis Os*	*Long gu*	2.5

This is a harmonizing sedative used for many psycho-neurological symptoms associated with agitation, as well as feelings of stagnation in the chest and upper abdomen; in short, it is used to treat true or false heat in the liver, which, in turn, has caused mental restlessness. It is effective in harmonizing the exterior and interior of the body, thus effecting a sedating effect on the mind. It is also a diuretic. The type of person this formula is frequently used for is yin weak and yang strong, a typical type A personality.

Functions:

Harmonizes interior and exterior, pacifies the spirit, and induces calm.

Main Conformations:

Irritable, easily frightened, insomniac, delirious, chest distress, resistance and distention beneath the heart with palpitations above the umbilicus, constipation, decreased urine, sensation of lassitude, and edema.

Major Indications:

1. Pulse; tense and rapid wiry.
2. Tongue; purple or red.
3. Abdomen; tight with resistance and distention in the hypochondriac area and palpations above the umbilicus.
4. Insomnia, hysteria, delirium, and neurosis.
5. Constipation and/or edema.
6. Hypertension and heart disease.
7. Epilepsy.
8. PMS symptoms.
9. Neurotic impotence/menopausal disorders.

References from the Classics:

Shang Han Lun, page 18. "The patient still suffering from a *shang han* condition eight to nine days after treatment with the purgation method, feeling fullness in the chest, anxiety and nervousness, dysuria, delirium, heaviness of the body, and difficulty in turning should be treated with *Chai hu jia long gu mu li tang* (Bupleurum and Dragon Bone Combination)."

Bupleurum and Hoelen Combination

Chai ling tang

Bupleurum	*Bupleuri Radix*	*Chai hu*	5.0
Pinellia	*Pinellia Tuber*	*Ban xia*	4.0
Scute	*Scutellariae Radix*	*Huang qin*	2.5
Ginseng	*Ginseng Radix*	*Ren shen*	2.5
Jujube	*Zizyphi Fructus*	*Da zao*	2.5
Ginger (fresh)	*Zingiberis Rhizoma*	*Sheng jiang*	4.0
Licorice	*Glycyrrhizae Radix*	*Gan cao*	2.0
Cinnamon Twigs	*Cinnamomi Ramulus*	*Gui zhi*	2.5
Polyporus	*Polyporus*	*Zhu ling*	2.5
Atractylodes (white)	*Atractylodis Rhizoma*	*Bai shu*	2.5
Hoelen	*Poria*	*Fu ling*	2.5
Alisma	*Alismatis Rhizoma*	*Ze xie*	4.0

This harmonizing formula is a combination of *Xiao chai hu tang* (Minor Bupleurum Combination) and *Wu ling san* (Hoelen Five Herb Combination). It is used for average type persons (usually women) with water/blood disorders affecting mainly liver and kidney energy. This generally manifests itself as stagnant blood and excess water in the lower jiao rising as heat into the middle and upper jiaos. Thus, the formula is particularly effective in treating gynecological disorders.

Functions:

Dispels stagnant water, strengthens spleen, and harmonizes and relieves lesser yang diseases.

Major Indications:

1. Pulse; varies greatly, can be wiry, slippery or moderate, and can also be rapid.
2. Tongue; flabby, purple or red, and can be red tipped, moist or dry.
3. Abdomen; water stagnancy in lower abdomen and lax.
4. Migraine headaches.
5. Menopausal symptoms.

6. Hypertension.
7. Edema.
8. Menstrual irregularities or difficulties.
9. Premenstrual syndrome (PMS).
10. Liver and gallbladder disorders.
11. Kidney disorders.

Cinnamon and Hoelen Formula

Gui zhi fu ling wan

Cinnamon Twigs	*Cinnamomi Ramulus*	*Gui zhi*	4.0
Hoelen	*Poria*	*Fu ling*	4.0
Persica	*Persicae Semen*	*Tao ren*	4.0
Peony	*Paeoniae Radix*	*Shao yao*	4.0
Moutan	*Moutan Radicis Cortex*	*Mu dan pi*	4.0

This is a blood moving formula which improves circulation and disperses blood stagnation. It warms lower body chill and water accumulations and rids internal heat from the upper body. It is used for persons with a strong constitution and a kidney type body. It can be used for acute flare-ups or chronic blood stagnation, which cause menstrual difficulty, and/or menstrual irregularity.

Functions:

Disperses stagnant blood and lumps in the abdomen.

Main Conformations:

Blood stagnation in the face and lips, cardiac hyperfunction, spasm in the left rectus abdominis muscle, lumps in lower abdomen weak pain on pressure, lower abdominal and low back pain, melena (evacuation resembling tar), and menstrual irregularity.

Major Indications:

1. Pulse; deep, tense, and slow.
2. Tongue; red, purple, and flabby.

3. Abdomen; tight with lumps and spasms.
4. Flushingup, headaches, and vertigo.
5. Arthritis, rheumatism, and neuralgia.
6. Endometriosis.
7. Menopausal symptoms.
8. Dysmenorrhea and PMS.
9. Hypertension, hysteria, and nervousness.
10. Eczema, dermatitis, pimples, and black spots.
11. Lumbago and shoulder pain.

References from the Classics:

Chin Kuei Yao Lueh, page 141. "Movement above the navel with sudden incessant uterine bleeding three months after the cessation of menses indicates the presence of a tumor. However, movement in the sixth month with regular menses in the first three months signals pregnancy. Blood discharged in the first three months is vicious (stagnant) blood, but should be discharged with *Gui zhi fu ling wan* (Cinnamon and Hoelen Formula)."

Bupleurum and Peony Formula

Jia wei xiao yao san

Tang-kuei	*Angelicae Radix*	*Dang gui*	3.0
Peony	*Paeoniae Radix*	*Shao yao*	3.0
Gardenia	*Gardeniae Fructus*	*Zhi zi*	2.0
Atractylodes (white)	*Atractylodis Rhizoma*	*Bai shu*	3.0
Hoelen	*Poria*	*Fu ling*	3.0
Mentha	*Menthae Herba*	*Bo he*	1.0
Bupleurum	*Bupleuri Radix*	*Chai hu*	3.0
Moutan	*Moutan Radicis Cortex*	*Mu dan pi*	2.0
Ginger (dried)	*Zingiberis Siccatum Rhizoma*	*Gan jiang*	1.0
Licorice	*Glycyrrhizae Radix*	*Gan cao*	2.0

This is a harmonizing formula used in situations where the liver overacts the spleen, and where it can nourish liver yin in average-strong persons. It has a broad spectrum of usage, which includes gynecological disorders, aching of the arms and legs, mental instability, flushingup, dizziness, insomnia, thirst, and abdominal distention; all of which are due to stagnant blood. The *Japanese Medical News* reports that this formula is the best remedy for cirrhosis, abdominal tenseness, thirst with a persistent and bitter taste in the mouth, turbid urine, and nosebleed. It is also very effective in the treatment of gynecological disorders due to stagnant blood in the lower jiao.

Functions:

Soothes liver, removes liver qi stagnancy, tonifies spleen and blood, purges excess fire, and regulates menstruation.

Main Conformations:

Cardiac hyperfunction, facial pallor, neurosis, insomnia, amnesia, coughing of blood, abdominal laxity, menstrual irregularity, hemorrhages including intestinal and uterine, urinary bleeding, and fatigue.

Major Indications:

1. Pulse; tight, tense, but empty and possibly deep.
2. Tongue; pale, purple, or red dots and may have red tip.
3. Abdomen; tight and distended.
4. Premenstrual syndrome (PMS) symptoms.
5. Irregular menses and infertility.
6. Menopausal symptoms.
7. Leukorrhea.
8. Constipation.
9. Acute and chronic damp heat infections.
10. Headaches and insomnia.
11. Mental disorders.

Gentiana Combination

Long dan xie gan tang

Gentiana	*Gentianae Scabrae Radix*	*Long dan*	1.0
Alisma	*Alismatis Rhizoma*	*Ze xie*	3.0
Akebia	*Akebiae Caulis*	*Mu tong*	5.0
Plantago	*Plantaginis Semen*	*Che qian zi*	3.0
Tang-kuei	*Angelicae Radix*	*Dang gui*	5.0
Rehmannia (raw)	*Rehmanniae Radix*	*Sheng di huang*	5.0
Gardenia	*Gardeniae Fructus*	*Zhi zi*	1.0
Scute	*Scutellariae Radix*	*Huang qin*	3.0
Licorice	*Glycyrrhizae Radix*	*Gan cao*	1.0

This is a fire purging formula which is used for persons of strong to average constitution; it is contraindicated in persons with a delicate constitution. It eliminates heat and inflammation, and should be administered only briefly. It is best for acute flare-ups of true heat signs, symptoms of liver yang rising and heat in the blood or damp/heat in the lower jiao. Symptoms include pain in the armpits, deafness, swollen ears, blood in the urine, and redness of the mouth and eyes.

Functions:

Clears liver heat and dampness.

Main Conformations:

Strong conformation, pale dark skin, tension and hypersensitivity on the outside of the abdominal rectus muscle, pain and swelling in the lower abdomen, and dampness on the inside of the hands and feet.

Major Indications:

1. Pulse; tense, rapid, forceful, and rolling.
2. Tongue; red with thick yellow coat.
3. Abdomen; tension, pain, and swelling in the lower abdomen.
4. Acute leukorrhea.
5. Gonorrhea and endometritis.
6. Hematuria, cystitis, and urethritis.

7. Herpes.
8. Itching, inflammation, and pain in genital area.
9. Eczema and orchitis.

Rhubarb and Leech Combination

Di dang tang

Leech	*Hirudo*	*Shui zhi*	1.0
Gadfly	*Tabanus*	*Meng chung*	1.0
Persica	*Persicae Semen*	*Tao ren*	1.0
Rhubarb	*Rhei Rhizoma*	*Da huang*	3.0

This is a blood moving formula which is very cooling and should be taken only briefly. Because it is so cooling, it is fast acting and aggressive; therefore, persons taking it need to be monitored very closely. This formula moves long standing stagnant blood, and is considered a *yang ming* formula due to its purging effect. It is used for treating symptoms such as lower abdominal distention with resistance and pain upon palpation, dark stools, polyuria, amnesia, and anxiety.

Functions:

Activates and regulates blood and disperses stagnant blood.

Major Indications:

1. Pulse; wiry and tight.
2. Tongue; purple, rigid, and red dots or bumps at the back of the tongue.
3. Abdomen; distended, painful, and tight.
4. Uterine myoma.
5. Dysmenorrhea and amenorrhea.
6. Dysuria and polyuria.
7. External injuries.

References from the Classics:

Shang Han Lun, page 19. "Greater yang disease that has lasted six or seven days, but which has not yet become a lesser yang condition, exhibiting residual surface symptoms, a feeble (superficial palpation), a sinking pulse (deep palpation), an absence of stagnancy in the chest, delirium due to fever in the lower jiao, hardness and fullness in the lower abdomen, and polyuria associated with blood stagnation may be cured by a discharge of blood, and should be given *Di dang tang* (Rhubarb and Leech Combination)."

Shang Han Lun, page 20. "Greater yang disease that exhibits a yellowish skin, sinking and knotted pulse, hardness of the lower abdomen, polyuria, and a manic state should be treated primarily with *Di dang tang* (Rhubarb and Leech Combination)...*Shang han* conditions of fever and fullness in the lower stomach, where there is dysuria instead of polyuria, should be purged and treated with *Di dang tang* (Rhubarb and Leech Combination)."

Shang Han Lun, page 40. "If a patient with sunlight yang conformation suffers from a loss of memory and has signs of stagnant blood and hard stools, but no difficulty in moving the bowels, he should be treated by the purgation method along with *Di dang tang* (Rhubarb and Leech Combination)."

Chin Kuei Yao Lueh, page 156. "A woman with scanty menses should take *Di dang tang* (Rhubarb and Leech Combination). This formula is also used to treat men's urinary bladder distention and urgency due to stagnant blood."

Persica and Rhubarb Combination

Tao he cheng qi tang

Persica	*Persicae Remen*	*Tao ren*	5.0
Rhubarb	*Rhei Rhizoma*	*Da huang*	3.0
Cinnamon twig	*Cinnamomi Ramulus*	*Gui zhi*	4.0
Mirabilitum	*Natrium Sulfuricum*	*Mang xiao*	2.0
Licorice	*Glycyrrhzeae Radix*	*Gan cao*	1.5

This formula is primarily used for treating stagnant blood in the lower jiao of strong constitution type persons. Generally speaking, such disease will be long standing, and since it is on a blood level, one will often see marked flushingup. This formula acts on a superficial level in treating toxins in the large intestine as well as heat in the liver; urogenital disorders due to stagnant blood are often seen here as well.

Functions:

Disperses stagnant blood and lumps in the abdomen.

Main Conformations:

Occluded blood, strong conformation, over excitability, hysteria, tinnitus with vertigo, dry mouth, flushingup with redness around the nose, general burning sensation, pulsation of the abdominal artery, sensation of distention in the lower abdomen, pain in the lower abdomen and lower back, constipation, spasms and coldness in the legs and feet, and uterine bleeding.

Major Indications:

1. Pulse; deep and tight, or floating.
2. Tongue; red or purple with yellow coat.
3. Abdomen; distention, cramping and pain in lower *jiao*, pain upon palpation, and pulsation of the abdominal artery.
4. Constipation.
5. Menstrual irregularities, dysmenorrhea, and menopausal symptoms.
6. Endometriosis and ovaritis.
7. Bleeding and hemorrhage.
8. Hypertension.
9. Emotional instability.
10. Skin disease due to heat in the blood.
11. Headache, vertigo, and tinnitus.
12. Low back pain.
13. Spasms and coldness in the hands and feet.

References from the Classics:

Shang Han Lun, page 18. "An unrelieved greater yang disease that exhibits a feverish lower jiao (the area between the stomach and the bladder) will result in extravasated blood which, in turn, will cause delirium in the patient. This condition may be helped by eliminating the extravasated blood from a bloody stool. However, if the surface symptoms do not improve, with or without the bloody stool, purgative herbs should not be further administered. The surface symptoms should be relieved first, and, when this is done, the acute lower abdominal pain may be dispersed with *Tao he cheng qi tang* (Persica and Rhubarb Combination)."

Lithospermum and Oyster Shell Combination

Zi gen mu li tang

Tang-kuei	*Angelicae Radix*	*Dang gui*	5.0
Peony	*Paeoniae Radix*	*Shao yao*	3.0
Cnidium	*Cnidii Rhizoma (Ligustici Rhizoma)*	*Chuan xiong*	3.0
Oyster Shell	*Ostreae Testa*	*Mu li*	4.0
Rhubarb	*Rhei Rhizoma*	*Da huang*	1.5
Cimicifuga	*Cimicifugae Rhizoma*	*Sheng ma*	2.0
Astragalus	*Astragali Radix*	*Huang qi*	2.0
Licorice	*Glycyrrhizae Radix*	*Gan cao*	1.0
Lonicera	*Lonicerae Flos*	*Jin yin hua*	1.5
Lithospermum	*Lithospermi Radix*	*Zi cao*	3.0

This formula is used for treating skin and lymph manifestations (e.g., recalcitrant swelling ulcers) associated with heat toxin in the blood. It is specific for treating skin cancer and breast cancer in weakened persons. Cancer is caused by chronic heat in the blood which leads to overall weakness in the person.

Functions:

Detoxifies blood, disperses hardness, and heals malignant sores.

Main Conformations:

Weak conformation, malignant skin disease, breast cancer, anemia, and lymphadenoma.

Major Indications:

1. Pulse; rapid, and empty, or weak.

2. Tongue; red with yellow coat.

3. Abdomen; without vital resistance.
4. Skin cancer.
5. Breast cancer.
6. Mastitis.
7. Lymphadenitis in the neck.
8. Gangrene in the lungs.

Lotus Seed Combination

Qing xin lian zi yin

Lotus Seed	*Nelumbonis Semen*	*Lian zi*	4.0
Ophiopogon	*Ophiopogonis Tuber*	*Mai men tong*	4.0
Hoelen	*Poria*	*Fu ling*	4.0
Ginseng	*Ginseng Radix*	*Ren shen*	3.0
Plantago	*Plantaginis Semen*	*Che qian zi*	3.0
Scute	*Scutellariae Radix*	*Huang qin*	3.0
Astragalus	*Astragali Radix*	*Huang qi*	2.0
Lycium Bark	*Lycii Radicis Cortex*	*Di gu pi*	2.0
Licorice	*Glycyrrhizae Radix*	*Gan cao*	2.0

This formula comes under the fire purging category, but it is important to realize that such heat is only in the upper jiao. Since the lower jiao is cold, the formula is designed not only to purge heat in the upper jiao, but also to harmonize the upper and lower jiaos; it nourishes the spleen, stomach and kidneys, and dispels internal heat in the heart and lungs. Persons taking this formula will be of delicate constitution, show heat rising, have chronic disorders, and general fatigue and weakness. The formula nourishes and regulates yin, including the fluid aspect of yin.

Functions:

Clears heart heat, dispels moisture, tonifies qi, nourishes yin, and supplements spleen and kidneys.

Main Conformations:

Excess symptoms in the upper part of the body and deficient

symptoms in the lower part of the body, nervousness, extreme thirst, bitter taste in the mouth, dry throat, discomfort in the heart, and tired arms and legs.

Major Indications:

1. Pulse; weak, rapid, and thready or slippery.
2. Tongue; pale, flabby, and dry or pasty (cotton mouth).
3. Abdomen; weak and flabby.
4. General fatigue.
5. Gastrointestinal weakness.
6. Chronic leukorrhea and gonorrhea.
7. Diabetes mellitus.
8. Anorexia.
9. Dysuria and cystitis.
10. Impotence.

Licorice and Jujube Combination

Gan mai da zao tang

Licorice	*Glycyrrhizae Radix*	*Gan cao*	5.0
Wheat	*Tritici Fructus*	*Fu xiao mai*	20.0
Jujube	*Zizyphi Fructus*	*Da zao*	6.0

This is a sedating formula which relaxes both the mind and the muscles of the body. Persons taking it will have a deficient constitution, and can be either lean and wiry or flabby and heavy, but will have a general lack of muscle tone and a susceptibility to pain.

Functions:

Nourishes the heart, pacifies the spirit, and relieves acute symptoms.

Main Conformations:

Despair and crying, excitability, insomnia, coma, hysteria, frequent yawning, general spasmodic muscles, and convulsions in the rectus abdominis muscle.

Major Indications:

1. Pulse; generally deep and deficient, although on a superficial level it can be rapid and tight/wiry.
2. Tongue; pale, quivering, possibly red tipped, and curving to one side.
3. Abdomen; tight with spasms.
4. Hysteria and neurosis.
5. Nervous exhaustion.
6. Insomnia, sleepwalking, and night cramps.
7. Epilepsy and chorea.
8. Gastrointestinal and uterine cramping and spasms.
9. Spasmodic cough.
10. Muscle spasms.

References from the Classics:

Chin Kuei Yao Lueh, page 152-153. "A woman with visceral irritation (hysteria) tends to grieve and cry as though possessed by a spirit. She also yawns frequently. She needs *Gan mai da zao tang* (Licorice and Jujube Combination)... This formula supplements splenic qi."

Ginseng and Longan Combination

Gui pi tang

Astragalus	*Astragali Radix*	*Huang qi*	2.0
Ginseng	*Ginseng Radix*	*Ren shen*	3.0
Hoelen	*Poria*	*Fu ling*	3.0
Atractylodes (white)	*Atractylodis Rhizoma*	*Bai shu*	3.0
Zizyphus	*Zizyphi Spinosi Semen*	*Suan zao ren*	3.0
Longan	*Longanae Arillus*	*Long yan rou*	3.0
Tang-kuei	*Angelicae Radix*	*Dang gui*	2.0
Ginger (dried)	*Zingiberis Siccatum Rhizoma*	*Gan jiang*	1.0
Jujube	*Zizyphi Fructus*	*Da zao*	1.0
Polygala	*Polygalae Radix*	*Yuan zhi*	1.0
Licorice	*Glycyrrhizae Radix*	*Gan cao*	1.0
Saussurea	*Saussureae Radix*	*Mu xiang*	1.0

This is a blood building and moving formula which is generally used for women with spleen/heart imbalance (i.e., deficient spleen robbing heart yin) affecting the qi and blood; this causes gastrointestinal weakness, menstrual irregularities, and insomnia. It can also be used for an acute or recent loss of blood which may cause overall debility. Persons for whom this formula is intended have weak constitutions.

Functions:

Tonifies qi, strengthens spleen, supplements blood, nourishes heart, and pacifies the spirit.

Main Conformations:

Cardiac hyperfunction, facial pallor, neurosis, insomnia, amnesia, coughing up blood, abdominal laxity, menstrual irregularity, hemorrhages including intestinal and uterine, urinary bleeding, and fatigue.

Major Indications:

1. Pulse; deep, thin, and weak.
2. Tongue; pale, no coat, and possibly flabby.
3. Abdomen; flabby and weak.
4. Irregular menses and postpartum weakness.
5. Amnesia, insomnia, fatigue, and nervous exhaustion.
6. Bleeding (due to spleen qi deficiency) and hemorrhage.
7. Talk about self excessively and obsessed with self.
8. Anemia, pale complexion, and anorexia.
9. Flabby and no muscle tone.
10. Excess perspiration and night sweats.
11. Leukemia and uterine carcinoma.
12. Endometritis and genital itching.
13. Impotence and chronic gonorrhea.

Chapter 11

TANG-KUEI FORMULAS FOR GYNECOLOGICAL DISORDERS

The following formulas are arranged in order from the stronger and more aggressive to the more nutritive. This order is not meant as an absolute, but rather as a basic guide to how the formulas can be arranged for treatment.

During the yang ming (third) stage of gynecological disorders, the following should be considered:

- Tang-kuei and Persica Combination
  (*Fu yuan huo xue tang*)

- Tang-kuei, Evodia, and Ginger Combination
  (*Dang gui si ni jia wu zhu sheng jiang tang*)

- Tang-kuei and Eight Herb Formula
  (*Ba wei dai xia tang*)

- Tang-kuei and Magnolia Formula
  (*Wu ji san*)

- Tang-kuei and Peony Formula
  (*Dang gui shao yao san*)

During the tai yin (fourth) stage of gynecological disorders, the following should be considered:

- Tang-kuei Four Combination
  (*Si wu tang*)
- Tang-kuei and Gardenia Combination
  (*Wen qing yin*)
- Tang-kuei and Gelatin Combination
  (*Jiao ai tang*)
- Tang-kuei and Ginseng Eight Combination
  (*Ba zhen tang*)
- Tang-kuei Sixteen Herb Combination
  (*Shi liu wei liu qi yin*)

During the shao yin (fifth) stage of gynecological disorders, the following should be considered:

- Tang-kuei and Evodia Combination
  (*Wen jing tang*)
- Tang-kuei and Gambir Combination
  (*Qi wu jiang xia tang*)

Tang-Kuei Formulas for Gynecological Disorders

Formula	Stage	Classification	Qi, Water Blood	Disorder	Patient Type
Tang-kuei and Persica C.	yang ming	blood	blood	acute	strong
Tang-kuei, Evodia and Ginger C.	yang ming/ tai yin	chill dispelling	blood/ water	acute/ chronic	weak
Tang-kuei and Eight Herb F.	yang ming	carbuncle dermatosis	qi blood	chronic	weak
Tang-kuei and Magnolia C.	jue yin/ yang ming	dual dissolving	qi/ blood	chronic	weak
Tang-kuei and Peony C.	yang ming	gynecological	blood	chronic	weak
Tang-kuei Four C.	tai yin	blood	blood	chronic	weak
Tang-kuei and Gardenia C.	tai yin	blood	blood	chronic	weak
Tang-kuei and Gelatin C.	tai yin	gynecological	blood	chronic	weak
Tang-kuei and Ginseng Eight C.	tai yin	tonic	qi/ blood	chronic	weak
Tang-kuei Sixteen C.	tai yin	qi	qi/ blood	chronic	medium
Tang-kuei and Evodia C.	shao yin/ jue yin	gynecological	blood	chronic	weak
Tang-kuei and Gambir C.	shao yin/ tai yin	blood	blood	chronic	weak

Tang-kuei and Persica Combination

Fu yuan huo xue tang

Bupleurum	*Bupleuri Radix*	*Chai hu*	12.0
Tang-kuei	*Angelicae Radix*	*Dang gui*	9.0
Carthamus	*Carthami Flos*	*Hong hua*	6.0
Licorice	*Glycyrrhizae Radix*	*Gan cao*	6.0
Persica	*Persicae Semen*	*Tao ren*	12.0
Rhubarb Trichosanthes	*Rhei Rhizoma*	*Da huang*	9.0
Root	*Trichosanthis Radix*	*Gua lou gen*	9.0
Anteater Scales	*Mantas Squama*	*Chuan shan jia*	9.0

This formula is used for the treatment of stagnant blood in strong type persons. Symptoms include severe pain and pain due to the swelling of external injuries. This is a very aggressive formula and should not be taken over a long period of time. It is also contraindicated during pregnancy.

Functions:

Activates blood, disperses stagnant blood, and soothes the liver.

Major Indications:

1. Pulse; tight, wiry, and rapid.
2. Tongue; purple or red dots.
3. Abdomen; tight and possibly immovable lumps.
4. Fibroid tumors.
5. Ovarian cysts and dysmenorrhea.
6. Absent, irregular, or interrupted menses or lactation.
7. Retained products of conception in women with true heat.
8. Constipation and hemorrhoids.
9. Dry skin.
10. Chest pain.
11. Blood toxins.

Tang-kuei, Evodia and Ginger Combination

Dang gui si ni jia wu zhu yu sheng jiang tang

Tang-kuei	*Angelicae Radix*	*Dang gui*	3.0
Cinnamon Twigs	*Cinnamomi Ramulus*	*Gui zhi*	3.0
Peony	*Paeoniae Radix*	*Shao yao*	3.0
Asarum	*Asari Herba Cum Radice*	*Xi xin*	2.0
Licorice	*Glycyrrhizae Radix*	*Gan cao*	2.0
Akebia	*Akebiae Caulis*	*Mu tong*	3.0
Jujube	*Zizyphi Fructus*	*Da zao*	5.0
Evodia	*Evodiae Fructus*	*Wu zhu yu*	2.0
Ginger (fresh)	*Zingiberis Rhizoma*	*Sheng jiang*	4.0

This is a chill dispelling formula which is used to treat chronic cold blood stagnation in the middle and lower jiaos. Symptoms include dysmenorrhea and other GYN situations where there is internal and external coldness and internal water poisoning. This formula warms the blood and improves overall blood circulation in weak persons. The usual body type of these individuals is obese.

Functions:

Warms the body and meridians, dispels cold, subdues ascending qi, and arrests vomiting.

Main Conformations:

Stagnant chills in the interior, cold sweats, annoying fullness in the chest, vomiting, abdominal spasm and pain, pain in the lower back, diarrhea, cold hands and feet (purple), asthma, and coughing up sputum.

Major Indications:

1. Pulse; thin, weak, and deep.
2. Tongue; flabby and pale.
3. Abdomen; pain and spasms.
4. Uterine bleeding and pain.
5. Dysmenorrhea.
6. Cold limbs and cold sweats.

7. Low back pain, sciatica, and cold nerve and joint disorders.
8. Diarrhea.
9. Calluses and corns.
10. Red spots on skin (petechia) and skin diseases.
11. Fatigue and anemia.

References from the Classics:

Shang Han Lun page 54. "*Dang gui si ni tang* (Tang-kuei and Jujube Combination) is recommended for patients with a sensation of chilled hands and feet (outside weakness of yang) and a small, weak pulse. This formula is given with *wu ji yu* (evodia) and *sheng qiang* (fresh ginger) when the patient exhibits prolonged chills on the inside in addition to the outside chills."

Tang-kuei and Eight Herb Formula

Ba wei dai xia fang

Tang-kuei	*Angelicae Radix*	*Dang gui*	5.0
Cnidium	*Cnidii Rhizoma (Ligustici Rhizoma)*	*Chuan xiong*	3.0
Hoelen	*Poria*	*Fu ling*	3.0
Akebia	*Akebiae Caulis*	*Mu tong*	3.0
Citrus	*Citri Leiocarpae Exocarpium*	*Chen pi*	2.0
Lonicera	*Lonicerae Flos*	*Jin yin hua*	1.0
Rhubarb	*Rhei Rhizoma*	*Da huang*	1.0
Smilax	*Smilacis Glabrae Rhizoma*	*Tu fu ling*	4.0

This formula is used for women of weak constitution who have damp heat symptoms such as leukorrhea with chronic constipation, mild anemia, subacute inflammation, and congestion. Such women may show signs of cold above and heat below. This formula is not as aggressive as *Long dan xie gan tang* (Gentiana Combination), but is used for similar indications. If a woman is showing signs of strong full heat, *Long dan xie gan tang* is recommended.

Functions:

Clears heat and moisture and treats leukorrhea.

Major Indications:

1. Pulse; weak.
2. Tongue; pale and yellow coat.
3. Abdomen; soft, weak, and congestion in lower areas.
4. Leukorrhea.
5. Urethritis.
6. Endometritis.
7. Itching and pain in the genital region.

Tang-kuei and Magnolia Formula

Wu ji san

Angelica	*Angelicae Dahuricae Radix*	*Bai zhi*	1.2
Citrus	*Citri Leiocarpae Exocarpium*	*Chen pi*	2.0
Cinnamon Twigs	*Cinnamomi Ramulus*	*Gui zhi*	1.2
Magnolia Bark	*Magnoliae Officinalis Cortex*	*Hou pu*	1.2
Tang-kuei	*Angelicae Radix*	*Dang gui*	1.2
Cnidium	*Cnidii Rhizoma (Ligustici Rhizoma)*	*Chuan xiong*	1.2
Peony	*Paeoniae Radix*	*Shao yao*	1.2
Hoelen	*Poria*	*Fu ling*	1.2
Platycodon	*Platycodi Radix*	*Jie geng*	1.2
Atractylodes (red)	*Atractylodis Lanceae Rhizoma*	*Cang shu*	4.0
Chih-ko	*Aurantii Fructus*	*Zhi ke*	1.2
Pinellia	*Pinellia Tuber*	*Ban xia*	2.0
Licorice	*Glycyrrhizae Radix*	*Gan cao*	1.2
Ginger (fresh)	*Zingiberis Rhizoma*	*sheng jiang*	1.2
Ma-huang	*Ephedrae Herba*	*Ma-huang*	1.2

This is a warming/harmonizing formula which aids in communication between the lungs, spleen, and kidney energies. Symptoms manifest mainly in the middle and upper jiaos, and affect the qi, water, and blood levels. There may be cold in the lower jiao, a delicate constitution and general weakness. This formula not only moves stagnant qi, water and blood, but tonifies as well; it is generally used for all three jiaos.

Functions:

Dispels accumulations of qi, blood, phlegm, cold, and food.

Main Conformations:

Sensation of fever in the upper part of the body and chills in the lower part, chilling pain and spasms in the waist and thighs, abdominal softness with diarrhea, facial anemia, headache, and vomiting.

Major Indications:

1. Pulse; sinking, weak, and possibly knotted or slippery.
2. Tongue; pale, flabby, and possibly red tipped.
3. Abdomen; lax and soft.
4. Menopausal symptoms.
5. Leukorrhea of the cold type.
6. Dysmenorrhea.
7. Aching at the waist and hernia.
8. Diarrhea.
9. Anemia.
10. Sensation of cold in lower body.
11. Chronic debility in postantibiotic states.
12. Acute and chronic gastroenteritis and gastric spasm.
13. Neuralgia and rheumatism.

Tang-kuei and Peony Formula

Dang gui shao yao san

Tang-kuei	*Angelicae Radix*	*Dang gui*	3.0
Peony	*Paeoniae Radix*	*Shao yao*	4.0
Hoelen	*Poria*	*Fu ling*	4.0
Atractylodes (white)	*Atractylodis Rhizoma*	*Bai shu*	4.0
Cnidium	*Cnidii Rhizoma* (*Ligustici Rhizoma*)	*Chuan xiong*	3.0
Alisma	*Alismatis Rhizoma*	*Ze xie*	4.0

This formula is used to move and warm blood in average to weak persons; it is suited mainly for women with blood stagnation due to weakness. It also addresses excess water affecting the stomach and/or kidney energy, making it very effective, then, in the treatment of postpartum weakness, general lassitude, menstrual disorders, ob/gyn related urinary tract problems, and infertility. It is specific in aiding women in carrying a fetus to full term, particularly if they have miscarried in the past.

Functions:

Tonifies blood and qi, activates blood, and promotes water metabolism.

Main Conformations:

Yin weakness conformation, chill conformation, irregular menstruation, prolonged menstrual flow, abnormal leukorrhea, lower abdominal and low back pain, rectus abdominis muscle spasms with softness of the abdominal wall, tinnitus, vertigo, heavy head, and anemia.

Major Indications:

1. Pulse; sinking, weak, and thready.
2. Tongue; pale, swollen, scalloped, and thin coat.
3. Abdomen; soft, painful with spasms of the rectus abdominis, and splashing sounds beneath the heart.
4. Body type; thin and soft muscles.
5. Leukorrhea.
6. Prolonged menstrual flow and irregular menses.
7. Anemia, fatigue, and pale and/or dry skin.
8. Edema, nephritis, and cystitis.
9. Increased or decreased urination.
10. Chills due to poor circulation.
11. Infertility and habitual abortion.
12. Postpartum weakness.
13. Tinnitus and vertigo.

References from the Classics:

Chin Kuei Yao Lueh, page 142. "*Dang gui shao yao san* (Tang-kuei and Peony Formula) helps pregnant women with abdominal cramping pain."

Chin Kuei Yao Lueh, page 157. "*Dang gui shao yao san* (Tang-kuei and Peony Formula) treats various women's abdominal problems."

Tang-kuei Four Combination

Si wu tang

Tang-kuei	*Angelicae Radix*	*Dang gui*	4.0
Peony	*Paeoniae Radix*	*Shao yao*	4.0
Cnidium	*Cnidii Rhizoma (Ligustici Rhizoma)*	*Chuan xiong*	4.0
Rehmannia (raw)	*Rehmanniae Radix*	*Di huang*	4.0

This formula is the base of all tang-kuei (dang gui) formulas. It is a very safe formula and is considered an "all purpose" formula for gynecological diseases. It builds and nourishes blood in overall blood deficient persons, and because of its blood building action, it also has a tranquilizing effect on the heart. It is considered a basic formula for anemia, weakness, or fever associated with blood loss or other blood deficiency. It is contraindicated in persons with deficient spleen yang causing diarrhea, gastrointestinal weakness, and severe anemia.

Functions:

Tonifies and activates blood; regulates menstruation.

Main Conformations:

Menstrual irregularity, uterine hemorrhage, hardening and pain in the lower abdomen, palpitation above the umbilicus, abdominal laxity, dry skin, anemia, and neurosis.

Major Indications:

1. Pulse; weak and thready.
2. Tongue; pale.

3. Abdomen; lax, with pain and hardness in the lower abdomen.
4. Amenorrhea and irregular menses.
5. Postpartum bleeding and weakness.
6. Abdominal pain in pregnancy.
7. Dry skin (due to deficient blood).
8. Uterine hemorrhage.
9. Weakness after abortion.
10. Intestinal or anal bleeding.

Tang-kuei and Gardenia Combination

Wen qing yin

Tang-kuei	*Angelicae Radix*	*Dang gui*	4.0
Rehmannia (raw)	*Rehmanniae Radix*	*Di huang*	4.0
Peony	*Paeoniae Radix*	*Shao yao*	3.0
Cnidium	*Cnidii Rhizoma (Ligustici Rhizoma)*	*Chuan xiong*	3.0
Coptis	*Coptidis Rhizoma*	*Huang lian*	1.5
Scute	*Scutellariae Radix*	*Huang qin*	3.0
Phellodendron	*Phellodendri Cortex*	*Huang bo*	1.5
Gardenia	*Gardeniae Fructus*	*Zhi zi*	2.0

This formula is for cooling, moving and building blood. It is used for weak-average type persons with chronic blood stagnation and damp heat, and it is a combination of *Si wu tang* (Tang-kuei Four Combination) and *Huang lian jie du tang* (Coptis and Scute Combination). The main signs for the use of this formula are areas of dark brown skin in various parts of the body. Bleeding skin, emotional disorders with internal heat, and liver blood deficiency symptoms can also be treated with this formula.

Functions:

Clears heat, cools, activates and disperses blood.

Main Conformations:

Uterine bleeding, ulcers on the external genitalia, dry itching skin, blackish, brown-yellow or brown skin, ulcers of the mouth, tongue and cheeks, neurotic excitability, and tension beneath the hypochondrium and rectus abdominis muscle.

Major Indications:

1. Pulse; rapid and tight or slippery.
2. Tongue; red, especially on the sides, and yellow coat.
3. Abdomen; tense--especially beneath the hypochondriac region and on the rectus abdominis muscle.
4. Liver disorders.
5. Uterine bleeding, menorrhagia, and metrorrhagia.
6. Hypertension.
7. Emotional instability.
8. Persistent leukorrhea.
9. Generalized skin diseases due to toxic heat (dermatitis, eczema, and urticaria).
10. Itching and dry skin.
11. Ulceration of the external genitals.
12. Ulceration of mouth, tongue, and cheeks--all membranes.
13. Peptic and duodenal ulcers.
14. Hemorrhage.

Tang-kuei and Gelatin Combination

Jiao ai tang

Tang-kuei	*Angelicae Radix*	*Dang gui*	4.0
Cnidium	*Cnidii Rhizoma (Ligustici Rhizoma)*	*Chuan xiong*	3.0
Peony	*Paeoniae Radix*	*Shao yao*	4.0
Licorice	*Glycyrrhizae Radix*	*Gan cao*	3.0
Artemisia	*Artemisiae Argyi Folium*	*Ai ye*	3.0
Rehmannia (raw)	*Rehmanniae Radix*	*Di huang*	5.0
Gelatin	*Asini Gelatinum*	*A jiao*	3.0

This is a tonic and a hemostatic formula which is specific for the treatment of acute hemorrhage. It not only stops bleeding, but also moves stagnant blood, strengthens overall weakness of the body resulting from excess bleeding, aids in the regulation of menstruation, and prevents miscarriage. It is effective for any type of person, but is contraindicated for individuals with fever and a flushed face.

Functions:

Tonifies and activates blood, regulates menstruation, stabilizes the fetus, and arrests uterine discharge.

Main Conformations:

Uterine bleeding, pain in the lower abdomen, melena (stools that resemble tar), annoying fever in the arms and legs, spasm of the left abdominis muscle, impairment of the lower abdomen, anemia, coughing or vomiting blood, and vertigo.

Major Indications:

1. Pulse; thready, empty, weak, and leek stalk.
2. Tongue; pale.
3. Abdomen; weak, painful, and spasms.
4. Uterine bleeding, endometritis, and uterine cancer.
5. Spotting midcycle.
6. Postpartum bleeding.
7. Menorrhagia.
8. Habitual abortion.
9. Intestinal or hemorrhoidal bleeding.
10. Weakness in arms and legs.
11. Anemia in weaker women.
12. Hemoptysis and hemopthalmia.

Tang-kuei and Ginseng Eight Combination

Ba zhen tang

Tang-kuei	*Angelicae Radix*	*Dang gui*	3.0
Rehmannia (cooked)	*Rehmanniae Radix*	*Shu di huang*	3.0
Cnidium	*Cnidii Rhizoma (Ligustici Rhizoma)*	*Chuan xiong*	3.0
Hoelen	*Poria*	*Fu ling*	3.0
Atractylodes (white)	*Atractylodis Rhizoma*	*Bai shu*	3.0
Licorice	*Glycyrrhizae Radix*	*Gan cao*	1.5
Peony	*Paeoniae Radix*	*Shao yao*	3.0
Ginseng	*Ginseng Radix*	*Ren shen*	3.0
Jujube	*Zizyphi Fructus*	*Da zao*	1.5
Ginger (fresh)	*Zingiberis Rhizoma*	*Sheng jiang*	3.0

This formula is a mixture of *Si wu tang* (Tang-kuei Four Combination) and *Si jun zi tang* (Four Major Herb Combination). It is used to treat general qi and blood deficiency, anemia with lack of vitality, liver and spleen weakness, underweight, severe chills and fever, coarseness of the skin, general weakness during convalescence, anorexia, lower abdominal distention, degeneration of the circulatory and digestive organs, and metrorrhagia during childbirth.

Functions:

Tonifies qi and supplements blood.

Main Conformations:

Irregular menstruation, distention in the lower abdomen (due to blood occlusion), lower back pain, degenerative digestive function, discomfort in the chest, fatigue and debility, extreme thirst, anemia, and loss of appetite.

Major Indications:

1. Pulse; weak and deep.
2. Tongue; pale and shaky.
3. Abdomen; distention due to blood occlusion.
4. Anemia.

5. Loss of appetite and extreme thirst.
6. Low back pain.
7. Fatigue and debility.
8. Irregular menstruation.

Tang-kuei Sixteen Herb Combination

Shi liu wei liu qi yin

Tang-kuei	*Angelicae Radix*	*Dang gui*	3.0
Cnidium	*Cnidii Rhizoma (Ligustici Rhizoma)*	*Chuan xiong*	3.0
Peony	*Paeoniae Radix*	*Shao yao*	3.0
Cinnamon Twigs	*Cinnamomi Ramulus*	*Gui zhi*	3.0
Ginseng	*Ginseng Radix*	*Ren shen*	3.0
Angelica	*Angelicae Dahuricae Radix*	*Bai zhi*	2.0
Platycodon	*Platycodi Radix*	*Jie geng*	3.0
Astragalus	*Astragali Radix*	*Huang qi*	2.0
Saussurea	*Saussureae Radix*	*Mu xiang*	2.0
Lindera	*Linderae Radix*	*Wu yao*	2.0
Magnolia Bark	*Magnoliae Officinalis Cortex*	*Hou pu*	2.0
Chih-ko	*Aurantii Fructus*	*Zhi ke*	2.0
Areca seed	*Arecae Semen*	*Bing lang*	2.0
Perilla Leaves	*Perillae Folium*	*Zi su ye*	2.0
Siler	*Ledebouriellae Radix*	*Fang feng*	2.0
Licorice	*Glycyrrhizae Radix*	*Gan cao*	2.0

This is a warming formula which is specific in the treatment of breast cancer, tumors, and intestinal diseases of unknown origin. It dissolves toxic tumors anywhere in the body, and not only breaks them up, but tonifies the body to combat further growth of tumors. It is used for average-weak constitutions.

Functions:

Tonifies and regulates qi and blood, and reduces swelling and pain.

Main Conformations:

Painful sores and tumors, breast cancer, goiter, and swelling of the lymph glands in the neck.

Major Indications:

1. Pulse; weak.
2. Tongue; pale.
3. Abdomen; weak and soft.
4. Breast cancer.
5. Fibrocystic disease.
6. Cervical lymphadenoma.
7. Painful tumors in the body.
8. Goiter.
9. Lymph gland swelling.
10. Intraductal papillomas.

Tang-kuei and Evodia Combination

Wen jing tang

Evodia	*Evodiae Fructus*	*Wu zhu yu*	1.0
Tang-kuei	*Angelicae Radix*	*Dang gui*	3.0
Cnidium	*Cnidii Rhizoma (Ligustici Rhizoma)*	*Chuan xiong*	2.0
Ginseng	*Ginseng Radix*	*Ren shen*	2.0
Cinnamon Twigs	*Cinnamomi Ramulus*	*Gui zhi*	2.0
Gelatin	*Asini Gelatinum*	*A jiao*	2.0
Moutan	*Moutan Radicis Cortex*	*Mu dan pi*	2.0
Ginger (dried)	*Zingiberis Siccatum Rhizoma*	*Gan jiang*	1.0
Peony	*Paeoniae Radix*	*Shao yao*	2.0
Licorice	*Glycyrrhizae Radix*	*Gan cao*	2.0
Pinellia	*Pinellia Tuber*	*Ban xia*	5.0
Ophiopogon	*Ophiopogonis Tuber*	*Mai men tong*	5.0

This formula is specific for the treatment of postpartum difficulty due to weakness. Such women will be deficient in both qi and blood, as well as cold in the lower jiao and have heat in the upper jiao. These will manifest as generally deficient liver yin, and deficient kidney yang causing weakness, flushingup, fever, thirst, and cold symptoms in the lower jiao. This formula is generally used for chronic cases in older women, but can also be used after a hysterectomy, or during pregnancy to prevent miscarriage.

Functions:

Tonifies and activates blood, warms the meridians, and regulates menstruation.

Main Conformations:

Irregular menstruation, prolonged menstrual flow, leukorrhea, annoying fever in the palms, sensation of distention and discomfort in the lower abdomen, lower back chills and pain, flushingup of qi, hiccups, and dry mouth and lips.

Major Indications:

1. Pulse; weak and deep.
2. Tongue; pale and dry.
3. Abdomen; painful, lax, discomfort, and distention in the lower abdomen.
4. Infertility.
5. Menopausal symptoms.
6. Chills in feet and groin area and feverish palms.
7. Irregular menses.
8. Leukorrhea (deficient type).
9. Habitual abortion and uterine bleeding.
10. Eczema, calluses, and corns.
11. Emotional disorders.

References from the Classics:

Chin Kuei Yao Lueh, page 154-155. "The disciples asked: Why would a woman of about fifty who had discharged blood for twenty to thirty days develop a fever at dusk, an urgent sensation in the lower abdomen, a full abdomen, an annoying fever in the palms, and dry lips?"

"The master answered: This is one of the diseases of exhaustion of the belt meridian. She has aborted and extravasated blood which has stagnated in the lower abdomen. How do we know this? Her dry lips tell the story. Treatment calls primarily for *Wen jing tang* (Tang-kuei and Evodia Combination). This formula aids women with chills in the lower abdomen and long term infecundity, metrorrhagia with loss of blood, and excessive or scanty menses."

Tang-kuei and Gambir Combination

Qi wu jiang xia tang

Tang-kuei	*Angelicae Radix*	*Dang gui*	3.0
Peony	*Paeoniae Radix*	*Shao yao*	3.0
Cnidium	*Cnidii Rhizoma (Ligustici Rhizoma)*	*Chuan xiong*	3.0
Rehmannia (raw)	*Rehmanniae Radix*	*Di huang*	3.0
Astragalus	*Astragali Radix*	*Huang qi*	3.0
Gambir	*Uncariae Ramulus Et Uncus*	*Gou teng*	4.0
Phellodendron	*Phellodendri Cortex*	*Huang bo*	2.0

This is a cooling formula which moves stagnant blood and water that is causing deficient yin symptoms. It is very effective in the treatment of hypertension due to kidney yin deficiency.

Functions:

Tonifies blood and qi, clears heat, and subdues liver tension.

Major Indications:

1. Pulse; rapid and thready.
2. Tongue; red and yellow coat.
3. Abdomen; tight with water stagnancy on the surface.
4. Essential hypertension.
5. Chronic nephritis.
6. Arteriosclerosis.
7. heaviness of the head.
8. Flushingup and tinnitus.
9. Aching shoulders.

Chapter 12

FEMALE VENEREAL DISORDERS

The following formulas are arranged in order from the stronger and more aggressive to the more nutritive. The order is not meant as an absolute, but rather a basic guide to how the formulas can be arranged for treatment.

During the shao yang (second) stage of female venereal disorders, the following should be considered:

- Cinnamon and Hoelen Formula
  (*Gui zhi fu ling wan*)

During the yang ming (third) stage of female venereal disorders, the following should be considered:

- Gentiana Combination
  (*Long dan xie gan tang*)

- Tang-kuei and Peony Formula
  (*Dang kuei shao yao san*)

During the tai yin and jue yin (fourth and sixth) stages of female venereal disorders, the following should be considered:

- Tang-kuei, Cinnamon and Peony Combination
  (*Dang gui jian zhong tang*)

- Cinnamon and Persica Combination
  (*Zhe chong yin*)

Female Venereal Disorder Symptoms

The following are basic disorders and indications commonly treated with the formulas in this section.

Chancroid

Symptoms: initial lesion at the site of inoculation in a macule or vesicopustule which soon breaks down to form a painful, soft ulcer with a necrotic base, surrounding erythema, and undermined edges. There may also be adenitis which is unilateral and consists of tender, matted nodes of moderate size, and overlying erythema.

Gonorrhea

Symptoms: external genitalia inflamed, reddened, moist and painful, and frequent and urgent urination may occur with a purulent urethral discharge.

Inguinal Bubo

Symptoms: pain in the groin area as a result of the inguinal lymph glands becoming swollen and red. There may be high fever, increasing pain, and eventually the formation of a pustule.

Syphilis

Symptoms: within two to three weeks after infection a local hard node, or chancre, forms. Skin eruptions in the form of pityriasis rosea, impetigo, and papules follow. Several months later syphilitic alopecia (patches of baldness) appear. Later rheumatic pain may be felt in the arms, and there may be rubber-like swellings, syphilitic leukorrhea, rubroderma, and ulcers.

Formulas for Female Venereal Disorders

Formula	Stage	Classification	Qi, Blood	Disorder	Patient Type
Cinnamon and Hoelen C.	shao yang	blood	qi/ blood	chronic	weak
Gentiana C.	yang ming	fire/ purging	blood	acute	strong
Tang-kuei and Peony C.	yang ming	gynecological	blood	chronic	weak
Tang-kuei, Cinnamon, and Peony C.	tai yin/ jue yin	chill dispelling	blood	chronic	weak
Cinnamon and Persica C.	jue yin	gynecological	blood	chronic	medium

Cinnamon and Hoelen Formula

Gui zhi fu ling wan

Cinnamon Twigs	*Cinnamomi Ramulus*	*Gui zhi*	4.0
Hoelen	*Poria*	*Fu ling*	4.0
Persica	*Persicae Semen*	*Tao ren*	4.0
Peony	*Paeoniae Radix*	*Shao yao*	4.0
Moutan	*Moutan Radicis Cortex*	*Mu dan pi*	4.0

This is a blood moving formula which circulates and disperses blood stagnation. It is used to warm the lower part of the body when there is cold due to water accumulation. It rids internal heat from the upper body, and is used for persons with a strong constitution and a kidney type body. It can be used when acute flare-ups or chronic blood stagnation causes menstrual difficulty and/or menstrual irregularity, as well as for female venereal diseases.

Functions:

Disperses stagnant blood and lumps from the abdomen.

Main Conformations:

Blood stagnation in the face and lips, cardiac hyperfunction, spasm in the left rectus abdominis muscle, lumps in lower abdomen (weak pain on pressure), lower abdominal and low back pain, melena (evacuation resembling tar), and menstrual irregularity.

Major Indications:

1. Pulse; deep, tense, and slow.
2. Tongue; red or purple, and flabby.
3. Abdomen; tight with lumps and spasms.
4. Flushingup, headaches, and vertigo.
5. Gonorrhea.
6. Endometriosis and PMS.
7. Menopausal symptoms.
8. Dysmenorrhea.
9. Leukorrhea.
10. Hypertension, hysteria, and nervousness.
11. Eczema, dermatitis, pimples, black spots, and urticaria.
12. Lumbago and shoulder pain.

References from the Classics:

Chin Kuei Yao Lueh, page 141. "Movement above the naval and sudden incessant uterine bleeding three months after cessation of menses indicates the presence of a tumor. However, movement in the sixth month with regular menses in the first three months signals pregnancy. Blood discharged in the first three months is vicious (stagnant) blood, but incessant uterine bleeding is due to a tumor which should be discharged with *Gui zhi fu ling wan* (Cinnamon and Hoelen Formula)."

Gentiana Combination

Long dan xie gan tang

Gentiana	*Gentianae Scabrae Radix*	*Long dan*	1.0
Alisma	*Alismatis Rhizoma*	*Ze xie*	3.0
Akebia	*Akebiae Caulis*	*Mu tong*	5.0
Plantago	*Plantaginis Semen*	*Che qian zi*	3.0
Tang-kuei	*Angelicae Radix*	*Dang gui*	5.0
Rehmannia (raw)	*Rehmanniae Radix*	*Sheng di huang*	5.0
Gardenia	*Gardeniae Fructus*	*Zhi zi*	1.0
Scute	*Scutellariae Radix*	*Huang qin*	3.0
Licorice	*Glycyrrhizae Radix*	*Gan cao*	1.0

This is a fire purging formula which is used for persons with a strong-to-average constitution, and is contraindicated in persons with a delicate constitution. The formula eliminates heat and inflammation, and should be administered only briefly. It is best for acute flare-ups of true signs and symptoms of liver yang rising, heat in the blood, or dampness/heat in the lower jiao. Symptoms include pain in the armpits, deafness, swollen ears, blood in the urine and redness of the mouth and eyes. In this application, it is used primarily for female venereal diseases where there is heat and dampness heat in the lower jiao.

Functions:

Clears liver heat and dampness.

Main Conformations:

Strong conformation, pale dark skin, tension and hypersensitivity on the outside of the rectus abdominis muscle, pain and swelling in the lower abdomen, and dampness on the inside of the hands and feet.

Major Indications:

1. Pulse; tense, rapid, forceful, and rolling.
2. Tongue; red with yellow coat.
3. Abdomen; tension, pain, and swelling in the lower abdomen.
4. Acute leukorrhea.

5. Gonorrhea.
6. Endometritis.
7. Hematuria.
8. Cystitis.
9. Urethritis.
10. Herpes and venereal ulcers.
11. Itching, inflammation, and pain in the genital areas.

Tang-kuei and Peony Formula

Dang gui shao yao san

Tang-kuei	*Angelicae Radix*	*Dang gui*	3.0
Peony	*Paeoniae Radix*	*Shao yao*	4.0
Hoelen	*Poria*	*Fu ling*	4.0
Atractylodes (white)	*Atractylodis Rhizoma*	*Bai shu*	4.0
Cnidium	*Cnidii Rhizoma (Ligustici Rhizoma)*	*Chuan xiong*	3.0
Alisma	*Alismatis Rhizoma*	*Ze xie*	4.0

This formula is used mainly for women with blood stagnation due to weakness. This includes postpartum weakness (and lassitude in general), tendency to miscarry, menstrual disorders, and infertility. A patient suffering from nausea, vomiting, and loss of appetite should not take this formula.

Functions:

Tonifies blood and qi, activates blood, and promotes water metabolism.

Main Conformations:

Yin weakness conformation, chill conformation, irregular menstruation, prolonged menstrual flow, abnormal leukorrhea, lower abdominal and low back pain, rectus abdominis muscle spasm with softness of the abdominal wall, tinnitus, vertigo, heavy head, and anemia.

Major Indications:

1. Pulse; deep and weak.
2. Tongue; pale and swollen.
3. Abdomen; painful and soft with spasms of the rectus abdominis muscle and splashing sounds beneath the heart.
4. Postpartum weakness.
5. Menstrual and pregnancy disorders.
6. Mold body, especially the feet.
7. Tinnitus and vertigo.
8. Gonorrhea.
9. Heaviness in the head.
10. Pale skin and anemia.
11. Chronic nephritis and cystitis.

References from the Classics:

Chin Kuei Yao Lueh, page 142. "*Dang gui shao yao san* (Tang-kuei and Peony Formula) helps pregnant women with abdominal cramping pain."

Chin Kuei Yao Lueh, page 157. "*Dang gui shao yao san* (Tang-kuei and Peony Formula) treats various women's abdominal problems."

Tang-kuei, Cinnamon and Peony Combination

Dang gui jian zhong tang

Peony	*Paeoniae Radix*	*Shao yao*	5.0
Tang-kuei	*Angelicae Radix*	*Dang gui*	4.0
Cinnamon Twigs	*Cinnamomi Ramulus*	*Gui zhi*	4.0
Ginger (fresh)	*Zingiberis Rhizoma*	*Sheng jiang*	4.0
Jujube	*Zizyphi Fructus*	*Da zao*	4.0
Licorice	*Glycyrrhizae Radix*	*Gan cao*	2.0

This is a formula used to treat those of delicate constitution who have anemia, continuous abdominal pain, bleeding, abdominal weakness, and abdominal spasms. Within this spectrum, this formula is beneficial to constitutionally weak woman who have venereal disease, especially acute or chronic PID (pelvic inflammatory disease).

Functions:

Warms stomach and spleen, supplements deficiency, and nourishes and harmonizes blood.

Main Conformations:

Generalized weakness, dragging pain in waist, back and legs, abdominal pain, labored breathing, loss of appetite, anemia, and melena (stools resembling tar).

Major Indications:

1. Pulse; weak and possibly rapid.
2. Tongue; pale.
3. Abdomen; soft and weak.
4. Peritonitis.
5. Uterine bleeding.
6. Abdominal pain.
7. Sciatica and lumbago.
8. Renal calculi and tubercular kidney.
9. Gonorrhea.

References from the Classics:

Chin Kuei Yao Lueh, page 149-150. "Postpartum feebleness and deficiency, incessant stabbing pain in the abdomen, difficult breathing, urgency in the lower abdomen with cramping pains extending to the lower back, and inability to eat and drink requires *Dang gui jian zhong tang* (Tang-kuei, Cinnamon and Peony Combination)."

Cinnamon and Persica Combination

Zhe chong yin

Moutan	*Moutan Radicis Cortex*	*Mu dan pi*	3.0
Cnidium	*Cnidii Rhizoma (Ligustici Rhizoma)*	*Chuan xiong*	3.0
Peony	*Paeoniae Radix*	*Shao yao*	3.0
Persica	*Persicae Semen*	*Tao-ren*	5.0
Cinnamon Twigs	*Cinnamomi Ramulus*	*Gui zhi*	3.0
Tang-kuei	*Angelicae Radix*	*Dang gui*	5.0
Carthamus	*Carthami Flos*	*Hong hua*	1.0
Corydalis	*Corydalidis Tuber*	*Yan husuo*	2.0
Achyranthes	*Achyranthis Radix*	*Niu xi*	2.0

This is a formula which is used for treating lower abdominal pain due to stagnant blood, pain in the pelvis, symptoms caused by stagnant blood during pregnancy, pelvic inflammatory disorder (PID), and venereal disease. For gonorrhea, this formula is used when symptoms are becoming chronic, and the inflammation is not serious.

Functions:

Tonifies and nourishes blood, disperses stagnant blood, and promotes the circulation of blood.

Main Conformations:

Blood occlusion in the lower abdomen, uterine myomatosis, pain in the lower abdomen, hemorrhage in the initial stage of pregnancy, and irregular or painful menstruation.

Major Indications:

1. Pulse; ropy.
2. Tongue; large red lumps in the rear of the tongue.
3. Abdomen; pain and lumpy stagnation.
4. Menstrual irregularities.
5. Peritonitis.
6. Uterine inflammation and ovaritis.
7. Miscarriage or spontaneous abortion.
8. Gonorrhea.

Chapter 13

MALE VENEREAL DISORDERS

The following formulas are arranged in order from the stronger and more aggressive to the more nutritive. The order is not meant as an absolute, but rather as a basic guide to how the formulas can be arranged for treatment.

During the tai yang (first) stage of male venereal disorders, the following should be considered:

- Ma-huang Combination
  (*Ma huang tang*)
- Coptis and Scute Combination
  (*Huang lian jie du tang*)
- Siler and Platycodon Formula
  (*Fang feng tong sheng san*)

During the yang ming (third) stage of male venereal disorders, the following should be considered:

- Rhubarb and Moutan Combination
  (*Da huang mu dan tang*)
- Gentiana Combination
  (*Long-dan-xie-gan-tang*)

- Polyporus Combination
  (*Zhu ling tang*)
- Croton and Hematite Formula
  (*Zi yuan*)

During the tai yin (fourth) stage of male venereal disorders, the following should be considered:

- Lotus Seed Combination
  (*Qing xin lian zi yin*)

Male Venereal Disorder Symptoms

Chancroid

Symptoms: initial lesion at the site of inoculation in the form of a macule or vesicopustule which soon breaks down to form a painful, soft ulcer with a necrotic base. This is surrounded by erythema with undermined edges. There may also be adenitis which is unilateral and consists of tender, matted nodes of moderate size with overlying erythema.

Gonococcal Prostatitis

Symptoms: acute prostatitis, perineal pain, fever, dysuria, frequent urination, urethral discharge, and enlarged prostate. Gentle palpation of the prostrate results in a copious purulent discharge.

Gonorrhea

Symptoms: initially burning on urination with a serous or milky discharge. One to three days later urethral pain becomes more pronounced, and the discharge becomes yellow, creamy and profuse, and is sometimes blood-tinged.

Inguinal Bubo

Symptoms: pain in the groin area due to the inguinal lymph glands becoming swollen and red. There may be a high fever and increasing pain, and eventually the formation of a pustule.

Syphilis

Symptoms: within two to three weeks after infection, a local hard node or chancre is formed. Skin eruptions in the form of pityriasis rosea, impetigo, and papules follow. Several months later syphilitic alopecia (patches of baldness) appears. Later on rheumatic pain may be felt in the arms, and there may be rubber-like swellings, syphilitic leukorrhea, rubroderma, and ulceration.

Formulas for Male Venereal Disorders

Formula	Stage	Classification	Qi, Water Blood	Disorder	Patient Type
Ma-huang C.	tai yang	sudorific	qi	acute	strong
Coptis and Scute C.	tai yang/ shao yang	fire purging	qi	acute	strong
Siler and Platycodon C.	tai yang/ yang ming	chronic	qi	dual dissolving	weak
Rhubarb and Moutan C.	yang ming	carbuncles dermatosis	blood	acute	strong
Gentiana C.	yang ming	fire/ purging	blood	acute	strong
Polyporus C.	yang ming	diuretic	water	acute	strong
Croton and Hematite C.	jue yin/yang ming	interior attacking	qi	acute	strong
Lotus Seed C.	tai yin	fire purging	water	acute	weak

Ma-huang Combination

Ma huang tang

Ma-huang	*Ephedrae herba*	*Ma huang*	5.0
Apricot Seed	*Armeniacae semen*	*Xing ren*	5.0
Cinnamon	*Cinnamomi ramulus*	*Gui zhi*	4.0
Licorice	*Glycyrrhizae radix*	*Gan cao*	1.5

This formula is used for treating common colds, headache, fever, general pain, and asthma in strong persons. Within these parameters, this formula is used in acute or recurrent/acute phase of venereal disease with aching and fever, but no perspiration.

Functions:

Relieves external symptoms, promotes sweating, promotes circulation of lung qi, and suppresses asthma.

Main Conformations:

Surface-fever-firm conformation, greater yang disease caused by wind cold invasion, generalized aching, and fever without sweating.

Major Indications:

1. Pulse; floating and tense.
2. Tongue; thin and white coat or normal.
3. Abdomen; firm.
4. Common cold with aching and fever, but no perspiration.
5. Upper respiratory infections.
6. Rheumatoid arthritis.
7. Cystitis.
8. Gonorrhea.

References from the Classics:

Shang Han Lun, page 9-10. "Greater yang disease with symptoms of headache, fever, generalized discomfort, low back pain, aching of the joints, mild chills, and gasping, but no perspiration, is treated with *Ma huang tang* (Ma-huang Combination)."

Shang Han Lun, page 11. "When greater yang disease with a floating and tense pulse, fever and generalized aching, but no perspiration has not improved after eight or nine days, it indicates that there is still a surface conformation, If the patient also suffers from anxiety and dizziness, and, in severe cases, epistaxis, *Ma huang tang* (Ma-huang Combination) is given. For the *shang han* condition associated with a floating and tense pulse, no perspiration, and a nosebleed should be treated primarily with *Ma huang tang* (Ma-huang Combination)."

Chin Kuei Yao Lueh, page 116. "Ma-huang, decocted in wine in winter and water in spring, treats jaundice."

Coptis and Scute Combination

Huang lian jie du tang

Scute	*Scutellariae Radix*	*Huang qin*	3.0
Coptis	*Coptidis Rhizoma*	*Huang lian*	1.5
Gardenia	*Gardeniae FRuctus*	*Zhi zi*	2.0
Phellodendron	*Phellodendri Cortex*	*Huang bo*	1.5

This is a heat clearing formula which is used to treat strong persons with true heat symptoms causing inflammation, anxiety, and bleeding. Generally it is used only in acute situations such as hemorrhage. It also is used for internal heat infections caused by liver fire.

Functions:

Clears heat, purges fire, arrests bleeding, and relieves irritability.

Main Conformations:

Yang strong conformation, cardiac hyperfunction, restlessness and insomnia, spitting and vomiting blood, facial reddening, chest discomfort with sensation of resistance beneath the heart, forceful abdomen, melena (stools resembling tar in appearance), and red urine.

Major Indications:

1. Pulse; forceful, deep, and rapid.
2. Tongue; red, possibly yellow coated, and possible bright red tip.
3. Abdomen; strong and tight.
4. Hypertension and anxiety.
5. Constipation.
6. Blood disorders.
7. Insomnia.
8. Resistance beneath the heart and palpitations.
9. Cerebral hemorrhage.
10. Gonorrhea.
11. Syphilis.
12. Herpes and urticaria.

13. Joint and nerve disorders.
14. Venereal disease with internal heat, inflammation, and bleeding.

Siler and Platycodon Combination

Fang feng tong sheng san

Tang-kuei	*Angelicae Radix*	*Dang gui*	1.2
Peony	*Paeoniae Radix*	*Shao yao*	1.2
Gardenia	*Gardeniae Fructus*	*Zhi zi*	1.2
Cnidium	*Cnidii Rhizoma (Ligustici Rhizoma)*	*Chuan xiong*	1.2
Forsythia	*Forsythiae Fructus*	*Lian qiao*	1.2
Ginger (fresh)	*Zingiberis Rhizoma*	*Sheng jiang*	1.2
Schizonepeta	*Schizonepetae Herba*	*Jing jie*	1.2
Siler	*Ledebouriellae radix*	*Fang feng*	1.2
Mentha	*Menthae Herba*	*Bo he*	1.2
Mirabilitum	*Natrium Sulfuricum*	*Mang xiao*	1.5
Ma-huang	*Ephedrae Herba*	*Ma huang*	1.2
Licorice	*Glycyrrhizae Radix*	*Gan cao*	2.0
Rhubarb	*Rhei Rhizoma*	*Da huang*	1.5
Atractylodes (white)	*Atractylodis Rhizoma*	*Bai shu*	2.0
Talc	*Talcum and Kaolinum*	*Hua shi*	3.0
Platycodon	*Platycodi Radix*	*Jie geng*	2.0
Scute	*Ledebouriellae Radix*	*Huang qin*	2.0
Gypsum	*Gypsum Fibrosum*	*Shi gao*	2.0

This is a formula which is good for strong full heat in both obese and non-obese constitutions. Symptoms include shoulder stiffness, numbness in the hands and feet, fatigue, headache, tight muscles, cardiac disorders, and habitual constipation. Within these categories, this formula is beneficial in treating overweight men with chronic venereal disease.

Functions:

Relieves exterior comformations and promotes sweating, purges interior heat and relieves constipation by dispelling the toxins of food, water and wind through the skin, excretory and digestive systems.

Main Conformations:

Obese constitution, facial reddening, yellowish white skin, constipation, and firmness and fullness in the abdomen which is centered at the umbilicus.

Major Indications:

1. Pulse; chordal, big, and strong.
2. Tongue; covered with bright red raised papillae.
3. Abdomen; firmness and fullness centered at the umbilicus.
4. Obesity.
5. Hypertension.
6. Arteriosclerosis.
7. Chronic nephritis.
8. Habitual constipation.
9. Skin diseases. (i.e., scabies and alopecia)
10. Arthritis.
11. Condyloma latum.
12. Gonorrhea.
13. Syphilis.

Rhubarb and Moutan Combination

Da huang mu dan pi tang

Rhubarb	*Rhei Rhizoma*	*Da huang*	2.0
Moutan	*Moutan Radicis Cortex*	*Mu dan pi*	4.0
Benincasa	*Benincasae Semen*	*Dong gua zi*	6.0
Mirabilitum	*Natrium Sulfuricum*	*Mang xiao*	4.0
Persica	*Persicae Semen*	*Tao ren*	4.0

This is a formula which is used for treating strong conformation persons who have a tendency towards constipation, fever, suppuration, and tumors in the lower abdomen. Within this spectrum, it is used for those with gonorrhea or venereal disease when it is suppurative in nature.

Functions:

Clears heat, disperses stagnant blood, disperses accumulations and hardness, and reduces carbuncles.

Main Conformation:

Strong conformation, tumor or hard lump in the lower abdomen, swelling pain and pain on pressure, fever in the abdomen, spontaneous sweating, frequent fever, and constipation.

Major Indications:

1. Pulse; tense and slow.
2. Tongue; red dots and bumps on the rear of the tongue.
3. Abdomen; palpable swelling and lumps, pain on pressure, and abdomen warm to the touch.
4. Colitis.
5. Proctitis.
6. Periproctitis.
7. Hemorrhoids.
8. Testitis.
9. Gonorrhea.
10. Leukorrhea.
11. Inguinal bubo.
12. Cystitis.

References from the Classics:

Chin Kuei Yao Lueh, page 134. "Lower abdominal swelling and hardening with aching upon pressure like that of urinary stuttering, normal urination, frequent fever, spontaneous sweating, and chillphobia which characterizes intestinal carbuncle. A slow and tense pulse indicates that pus has not yet developed. The condition may be treated by purgation which will cause bleeding. If the patient's pulse is surging and quick, pus has developed and the condition should not be treated by purgation, but with *Da huang mu dan tang* (Rhubarb and Moutan Combination)... If pus is present in the body, it will be discharged; if there is none, blood will be discharged."

Gentiana Combination

Long dan xie gan tang

Gentiana	*Gentianae Scabrae Radix*	*Long dan*	1.0
Alisma	*Alismatis Rhizoma*	*Ze xie*	3.0
Akebia	*Akebiae Caulis*	*Mu tong*	5.0
Plantago	*Plantaginis Semen*	*Che qian zi*	3.0
Tang-kuei	*Angelicae Radix*	*Dang gui*	5.0
Rehmannia (raw)	*Rehmanniae Radix*	*Sheng di huang*	5.0
Gardenia	*Gardeniae fructus*	*Zhi zi*	1.0
Scute	*Scutellariae radix*	*Huang qin*	3.0
Licorice	*Glycyrrhizae radix*	*Gan cao*	1.0

This is a fire purging formula which is used for persons with a strong to average constitution. It is condraindicated in persons with a delicate constitution. The formula eliminates heat and inflammation and should be administered only briefly. It is best for acute flare-ups of true heat signs and symptoms of liver yang raising, heat in the blood, or damp-heat in the lower jiao. Symptoms include pain in the armpits, deafness, swollen ears, blood in the urine and redness of the eyes. Within this spectrum, this formula will primarily be used for male venereal disease where there is heat or damp heat in the lower jiao.

Functions:

Clears liver heat and dampness.

Main Conformations:

Strong conformation, pale dark skin, tension and hypersensitivity on the outside of the abdominal rectus muscle, pain and swelling in the lower abdomen, and dampness on the inside of the hands and feet.

Major Indications:

1. Pulse; tense, rapid, forceful, and rolling.
2. Tongue; red and thick yellow coat.
3. Abdomen; tension, pain, and swelling in the lower abdomen.
4. Acute leukorrhea.

5. Gonorrhea and venereal ulcers.
6. Hematuria.
7. Cystitis.
8. Urethritis.
9. Herpes.
10. Itching, inflammation, and pain in genital area.
11. Eczema and orchitis.
12. Groin lymphadenitis.
13. Inguinal bubo.

Polyporus Combination

Zhu ling tang

Polyporus	*Polyporus*	*Zhu ling*	3.0
Hoelen	*Poria*	*Fu ling*	3.0
Alisma	*Alismatis Rhizoma*	*Ze xie*	3.0
Talc	*Talcum and Kaolinum*	*Hua shi*	3.0
Gelatin	*Asini Gelatinum*	*A jiao*	3.0

This is a formula which is diuretic and is used to treat urinary difficulties, lower abdominal tension and fever, thirst, fever, vomiting, anxiety, and insomnia by moistening dryness and dispelling fever. Within this spectrum, it is primarily used for male venereal disease with urinary, and possible, bleeding manifestations, as well as diagnosed kidney involvement.

Functions:

Nourishes yin and dispels water stagnancy.

Main Conformations:

Decreased urine, urinary stuttering pain, painful urination, edema, diarrhea, tension in the lower abdomen (toxic fever), discomfort in the chest with flushingup of qi, fever, extreme thirst neurosis, and insomnia.

Major Indications:

1. Pulse; floating and rapid.
2. Tongue; red/dry and possibly with dark yellow fur.
3. Abdomen; tension, fullness, and pain in lower abdomen.
4. Nephritis, urethritis, cystitis, and pyelitis.
5. Gonorrhea.
6. External or internal bleeding.
7. Edema.
8. Diarrhea.
9. Gonococcal prostatitis.

References from the Classics:

Shang Han Lun, page 38. "*Zhu ling tang* (Polyporus Combination) is recommended for patients with thirst and dysuria."

Shang Han Lun, page 50. "Patients with lesser yin disease characterized by persistent diarrhea for six to seven days, cough, vomiting, thirst, anxiety, and insomnia should be treated with *Zhu ling tang* (Polyporus Combination) in order to moisten the dryness and dispel the fever."

Chin Kuei Yao Lueh, page 9. "To treat visceral disease, prescribe a formula in accordance with the whole condition. For instance, if a person is thirsty, the formula *Zhu ling tang* (Polyporus Combination) will quench his thirst. This rule applies to all conditions."

Chin Kuei Yao Lueh, page 96. "A patient with a floating pulse, fever, thirst for water, and oliguria should be treated essentially with *Zhu ling tang* (Polyporus Combination)."

Croton and Hematite Formula

Zi yuan

Croton	*Semen Crotonis*	*Ba dou*	4.0
Hematite	*Haematitum*	*Dai zhe shi*	4.0
Kaolin	*Halloysitum Rubrum*	*Chi shi zhi*	4.0
Apricot Seed	*Armeniacae Semen*	*Xing ren*	8.0

This is a cathartic formula which is used for treating distention in the chest and abdomen. It acts fast to alleviate acute symptoms of gonorrhea during the initial stage in strong patients. Children with congenital syphilis having head abscesses and skin symptoms can also be treated with this formula.

Functions:

Purges and warms the body.

Main Conformations:

Fullness in the chest and abdomen due to water and food toxins and constipation

Major Indications:

1. Pulse; slippery.
2. Tongue; swollen and possibly aching.
3. Abdomen; fullness on palpitation.
4. Acute gastroenteritis, dysentery, and food poisoning.
5. Uremia.
6. Meningitis.
7. Paralytic ileus.
8. Constipation.
9. Gonorrhea.
10. Congenital syphilis.

Lotus Seed Combination

Qing xin lian zi yin

Lotus seed	*Nelumbonis Semen*	*Lian zi*	4.0
Ophiopogon	*Ophiopogonis Tuber*	*Mai men dong*	4.0
Hoelen	*Poria*	*Fu ling*	4.0
Ginseng	*Ginseng Radix*	*Ren shen*	3.0
Plantago	*Plantaginis Semen*	*Che qian zi*	3.0
Scute	*Scutellariae Radix*	*Huang qin*	3.0
Astragalus	*Astragali Radix*	*Huang qi*	2.0
Lycium bark	*Lycii radicis Cortex*	*Di gu pi*	2.0
Licorice	*Glycyrrhizae Radix*	*Gan cao*	2.0

This formula comes under the fire purging category, but it is important to realize that the heat treated is only in the upper jiao. The lower jiao will be cold, therefore, this formula is designed to harmonize the upper and lower regions of the body. It nourishes spleen, stomach and kidney, and dispels internal heat in the heart and lungs. Persons taking this formula should show signs of heat rising. Within this category, persons will have chronic gonorrhea or other forms of venereal disease with general fatigue and weakness. This formula nourishes and regulates the yin (cooling and moistening aspect of the body).

Functions:

Clears heart heat, dispels moisture, tonifies qi, nourishes yin, and supplements spleen and kidneys.

Main Conformations:

Excess symptoms in upper part of the body and deficient symptoms in lower part of the body, nervousness, extreme thirst, bitter taste in the mouth, dry throat, discomfort in the heart, and tired arms and legs.

Major Indications:

1. Pulse; weak, rapid, and thready or slippery.
2. Tongue; pale, flabby, dry, or pasty (cotton mouth).
3. Abdomen; weak, sloshing sounds, or flabby.
4. General fatigue.
5. Gastrointestinal weakness.
6. Chronic leukorrhea.
7. Gonorrhea.
8. Diabetes mellitus.
9. Anorexia.
10. Dysuria.
11. Cystitis.
12. Kidney disorders.
13. Impotence.
14. Gonococcal prostatitis.

INDIVIDUAL HERBS
(Materia Medica)

Akebia

(*Mu tong*, Akebiae Caulis)

Part Used: stem.

Essence and Flavor: bitter, and cold.

Channels Entered: heart, small intestine, and urinary bladder.

Functions:

1. Diuretic, and promotes water metabolism.
2. Antiinflammatory, and clears heat.
3. Promotes menstrual flow, and increases lactation.
4. Promotes blood circulation.

Medicinal Uses:

1. Acute UTI, and urinary calculus.
2. Edema, and urinary bladder dysfunction.
3. Amenorrhea, scanty lactation, and cramps.
4. Rheumatic arthritis.
5. Irritability and heat sensation in chest.
6. Sore throat and laryngitis.
7. Hematuria, and anemia.

Contraindications: persons with spermatorrhea, frequent urination, *xu qi*, dehydration, and pregnancy.

Anemarrhena

(*Zhi mu*, Anemarrhenae Rhizoma)

Parts Used: root.

Essence and Flavor: bitter, and cold.

Channels Entered: lung, stomach, and kidney.

Functions:

1. Removes heat, and purges fire in lungs and stomach.
2. Nourishes kidneys.
3. Moistens dryness--especially in lung.

Medicinal Uses:

1. Diabetes.
2. Cough due to fatigue.
3. Fevers, dryness, and heat.
4. Dysuria, tenesmus, and urinary disturbances due to heating.
5. Low back pain.
6. Chronic low grade febrile diseases, TB, and chronic bronchitis.

Contraindications: those with diarrhea.

Astragalus

(*Huang qi*, Astragali Radix)

Part Used: root.

Essence and Flavor: sweet, and warm.

Channel Entered: spleen, and lung.

Functions:

1. Tonifies qi and *wei qi*, and increases yang.
2. Tonifies the spleen.
3. Stabilizes the exterior, and stops sweating.
4. Promotes urination, and removes edema.
5. Discharges pus.

Medicinal Uses:

1. Lack of vigor.
2. Prolapse.
3. Spontaneous sweating.
4. Wasting and thirsting syndromes.

Contraindications: Persons with deficient yin or external heat patterns

Bupleurum

(*Chai hu*, Bupleuri Radix)

Part Used: root.

Essence and Flavor: slightly cold, and bitter.

Channel Entered: liver, gallbladder, pericardium, and triple warmer (jiao).

Functions:

1. Used as antipyretic for intermittent fever.
2. Relieves stagnancy of vital energy of the liver.
3. Elevates the vital energy of the spleen.
4. Resolves surface.
5. Disperses heat.

Medicinal Use:

1. Malaria; alternating chills and fever, and vomiting.
2. Pain in chest and hypochondriac area.
3. Visceroptosis.
4. Jaundice.
5. Deafness, and dizziness.

Contraindications: persons with excessive fire of the liver or deficiency of yin.

Cinnabar

(*Zhu xia*, Cinnabaris)

Part Used: mineral.

Essence and Flavor: sweet, cold, and toxic.

Channel Entered: heart.

Functions:

1. Sedative, and tranquilizer.
2. Anticonvulsive, and detoxicant.

Medicinal Uses:

1. Insomnia, and palpitations.
2. Epilepsy.
3. Infantile convulsions due to high fever.
4. Boils, furuncles, and carbuncles.

Contraindications: no true heat symptoms.

Cinnamon Bark

(*Gui pi*, Cinnamomi Cortex)

Part Used: bark.

Essence and Flavor: pungent, and warm.

Channel Entered: heart, liver, spleen, and kidney.

Functions:

1. Warm the spleen and stomach.
2. Dispel cold, and relieve pain.
3. Invigorate the circulation of blood.

Medicinal Use:

1. Gastrointestinal pain due to cold.
2. Lumbago, and arthralgia.
3. Anemia.

4. Spontaneous sweating.

Contraindications: pregnant women, and persons with deficiency of yin, or with excess fire and internal heat symptoms.

Cinnamon Twigs

(*Gui zhi*, Cinnamomi Ramulus)

Part Used: twig.

Essence and Flavor: sweet, and warm.

Channel Entered: lung, urinary bladder, and heart.

Functions:

1. Diaphoretic.
2. Warm the channels and collaterals.
3. Promote the circulation of *yang chi* in the chest.
4. Promote blood circulation.

Medicinal Use:

1. Common cold, and affection due to wind and cold.
2. Chest pain, palpitations, and angina pectoralis.
3. Edema, dysuria, and abdominal fullness.
4. Arthritic pain.
5. Amenorrhea.

Contraindications: persons with febrile disease, excess heat and fire, and pregnant women.

Clematis

(*Wei ling xian*, Clematidis Radix)

Part Used: root.

Essence and Flavor: pungent, salty, and warm.

Channel Entered: urinary bladder.

Functions:

1. Antirheumatic, and dispel wind and dampness.

2. Invigorate circulation of qi in all channels, and control pain.
3. Regulate urination.

Medicinal Uses:

1. Rheumatic pain in the whole body.
2. Fish bone stuck in throat feeling.
3. Gout, and pain in loins, knees and limbs.
4. Migraines.
5. Edema, and mass in abdomen.

Contraindications: spasms caused by *xu* blood.

Coix

(*Yi yi ren*, Coicis Semen)

(Job's Tears, Wild Barley)

Part Used: seed.

Essence and Flavor: sweet or no taste, and neutral or slightly cold.

Channel Entered: spleen, stomach, lung, and large intestine.

Functions:

1. Resolve dampness, and regulate water metabolism (osmotic diuretic).
2. Eliminate inflammation, and discharge pus.
3. Tonify spleen, and arrest diarrhea.
4. Relieve spasms and arthritic pain.
5. Benefit skin.

Medicinal Uses:

1. Edema, oliguria, tinea of foot, and ascites.
2. Lung and intestinal abscess.
3. Diarrhea.
4. Rheumatic arthritis.

Contraindications: pregnant women.

Pharmaceutical Action:

1. Action on striated muscles and motor nerve endings, excitatory action at low concentration, and paralysis at high concentration.
2. Excitatory action on frog heart, intestines, respiration, uterus, and skeletal muscles at small dosage, but inhibitory at large dosage.
3. Antidiuretic.
4. Antitumor.
5. Analgesic.
6. Antipyretic.

Coptis

(*Huang lian*, Coptidis Rhizoma, Golden Seal)

Part Use: root.

Essence and Flavor: bitter, and cold.

Channel Entered: heart, liver, stomach, gallbladder, and large intestine.

Function:

1. Eliminate heat and dampness.
2. Sedative.
3. Antitoxin, and detoxify fire poison.
4. Stop bleeding.
5. Drain stomach fire.

Medicinal Uses:

1. Digestive dysfunction, diarrhea, acute enteritis, and dysentery.
2. Insomnia, fidget, and delirium due to high fever.
3. Inflammation of mouth, tongue and throat.
4. Leukemia, conjunctivitis, and otitis media.
5. Sores, carbuncles, and abscesses.

Contraindications: deficient yin, and cold spleen, stomach and kidney.

Evodia

(*Wu zhu yu*, Evodiae Fructus)

Part Used: fruit.

Essence and Flavor: pungent, bitter, hot, and slightly toxic.

Channel Entered: spleen, stomach, liver, and kidney.

Function:

1. Warm spleen and stomach, and dispel cold.
2. Relieve pain.
3. Reverse the flow of qi.

Medicinal Uses:

1. Cold sensation in the stomach, gastralgia, and abdominal pain.
2. Vomiting, and acid regurgitation.
3. Diarrhea in the morning.

Contraindications: persons with deficiency of yin (vital essence), and excess fire.

Caution: overuse will cause dysopsia (visual disturbances), and illusions.

Pharmaceutical Action:

1. Antibacterial.
2. Antiparasitic.
   a. Pork tapeworm (teania solium).
   b. Pinworm (enterobius vermicularis).
3. Analgesic.
4. Increase body temperature.
5. Mild stimulation of respiration and blood pressure.
6. Contraction of uterus.
7. Action on the central nervous system--large dosage produces excitatory action, and may cause illusions and dysopsia.

Evodiamine:

1. Analgesic.
2. Mild stimulation of respiration and blood pressure.

Forsythia

(*Lian qiao*, Forsythiae Fructus)

Part Used: fruit.

Essence and Flavor: bitter, and slightly cold.

Channel Entered: lung, heart, and gallbladder.

Function:

1. Eliminate pathogenic heat and toxin from the blood.
2. Resolve abscess and disperse lumps and hardenings (antipyretic and antiinflammatory).

Medicinal Uses:

1. Common cold, and febrile disease.
2. High fever with thirst and delirium.
3. Urinary tract infection.
4. Scrofula and abscess.
5. Allergenic purpura.

Contraindication: persons with diarrhea, heat caused by deficiency of yin, or chronic purulent abscess.

Pharmaceutical Action:

1. Antibacterial (broad-spectrum)--inhibits the growth of Staph. areus, Shigella dysenteriae, hemolytic streptococcus, pneumonia, B. typhi, virus, Mycobacterium tuberculi, etc.
2. Antiemetic:
   a. Suppresses vomiting caused by digitalis and apomorphine.
   b. Inhibits emetic receptive center of the medulla oblongata.
3. Lower SGPT.
4. Excitatory action on the central nervous system.
5. Oleanolic acid acts as diuretic and cardiotonic.

6. Vitamin P can decrease vascular permeability and fragility, and prevent the effusion of blood.

Fritillaria

(*Bai mu*, Fritillariae Bulbus)

Part Used: bulb.

Essence and Flavor: bitter, sweet, and slightly cold.

Channel Entered: lung, and heart.

Functions:

1. Resolves phlegm, and relieves cough.
2. Nourishes and moistens lungs.
3. Disperses lumps and hardening.

Medical Uses:

1. Dry cough, and cough with little phlegm.
2. Chronic bronchitis.
3. TB.
4. Lung and breast abscess.
5. Goiter, and scrofula.

Contraindications: cold-damp phlegm in spleen and stomach.

Fritillaria

(*Bei mu*, Fritillariae Bulbus)

Part Used: bulb.

Essence and Flavor: bitter, and mildly cold.

Channels Entered: lung, and heart.

Functions:

1. Moisten dryness to resolve phlegm.
2. Control cough.
3. Clear heat.
4. Disperse lumps and hardenings.

Medicinal Uses:

1. Cough with thick sputum.
2. Acute bronchitis.
3. Pneumonia.
4. Subcutaneous.
5. Scrofula, and goiter.

Contraindications: cold/damp phlegm in spleen and stomach.

Gambir

(*Diao teng gou*, Gambir Vine)

(Uncariae Ramulus et Uncus)

Part Used: stem.

Essence and Flavor: sweet, and slightly cold.

Channels Entered: liver, pericardium, and heart.

Functions:

1. Anticonvulsant--reduce endogenous wind of liver, and relieve convulsions.
2. Antipyretic--clear heat in the liver.
3. Antihypertensive.

Medicinal Uses:

1. Convulsions with high fever.
2. Vertigo, and nervous and hypertensive headache.
3. Hypertension.

Contraindications: persons with no true heat or endogenous wind symptoms.

Pharmaceutical Action:

1. Sedative, but not hypnotic--lowers the excitation of the cerebral cortex, destroys some positive conditioned reflexes, and prolongs the time of the conditioned reflexes.

2. Antiepileptic--may cause motor paralysis and inhibition of respiration.

3. Antihypertensive:

a. If the decoction is boiled too long or not enough, the antihypertensive action is influenced. The best time for boiling is within 15 minutes.
b. By reflex, through the vagus nerve into the fiber, and inhibits the vascular motor center.
c. Dilation of blood vessels in rabbit's ears.
d. Significant effect on renal hypertension.

Gelatin

(*A jiao*, Asini Gelatinum)

Part Used: derived from processed skin of horse, cow or bull.

Essence and Flavor: sweet, and neutral.

Channels Entered: lung, liver, and kidney.

Function:

1. Nourish the blood.
2. Hemostatic--for bleeding of all kinds.
3. Nourish the yin.
4. Smooth the lung.

Medicinal Uses:

1. Anemia.
2. Hemoptysis, epistaxis, hematuria, and uterine bleeding.
3. Irritability, and paralysis.
4. Dry cough with bloody sputum, and tuberculosis.

Contraindications: persons with weak stomachs, and digestive disorders.

Gentiana

(*Long dan*, Gentianae Scabre Radix)

Part Used: root.

Essence and Flavor: bitter, and cold.

Channels Entered: liver, gallbladder, and stomach.

Functions:

1. Eliminate heat and dampness.
2. Sedate liver fire.

Medicinal Uses:

1. Jaundice, leukorrhea, and eczema.
2. Bloodshot eyes, conjunctivitis, sore throat, bitterness in mouth, and pain in the ear.
3. Acute infection of urinary system.
4. Hypertension with dizziness and tinnitus.

Contraindications: persons without true heat, fire or dampness symptoms.

Gypsum

(*Shi gao*, Calcium Sulfate, Gypsum Fibrosum)

Essence and Flavor: pungent, sweet, and very cold.

Channels Entered: lung and stomach.

Function:

1. Clear heat in the qi portion.
2. Clear heat in the lung and stomach.
3. Sedate fire, and relieve thirst.

Medicinal Uses:

1. High fever, fidget, and thirst.
2. Asthma caused by heat in the lung.
3. Headache, and gingivitis.

4. Burns, abscesses, and eczema.

Contraindications: persons with a weak stomach or stomach without true heat and dampness symptoms.

Hoelen

(*Fu-ling*, Tuckahoe, Indian Bread, Poria)

Part Used: sclerotium of the fungus.

Essence and Flavor: sweet, no taste, or neutral.

Channel Entered: heart, lung, spleen, stomach, and kidney.

Function:

1. Regulates water metabolism and resolves dampness (diuretic).
2. Reinforces the spleen and stomach.
3. Pacifies the heart (sedative), and soothes the nerves.
4. Harmonizes the middle warmer (jiao).

Contraindications: persons with polyuria, spermatorrhea, or prolapse of urogenital organs.

Licorice

(*Gan cao*, Glycyrrhizae Radix)

Part Used: root.

Essence and Flavor: sweet, and neutral.

Channel Entered: lung, spleen, and stomach.

Function:

1. Invigorate the function of the energy.
2. Clear pathogenic heat, and detoxify drug poisoning.
3. Spasmolytic, and relief of pain.
4. Antitussive, and expectorant.
5. Moderate the action of other herbs.

Medicinal Uses:

1. Palpation, weakness, and malaise due to qi deficiency.

2. Sore throat, boils, and carbuncles.
3. Cough, and asthma.
4. Peptic ulcer.
5. Addison's disease.

Contraindications: persons with fullness of the abdomen (*Shi*-excess syndrome).

Longan

(*Long yan hua*, Longanae Arillus)

Part Used: aril.

Essence and Flavor: sweet, and warm.

Channel Entered: heart, and spleen.

Functions:

1. Nourish blood, sedate, and stabilize the spirit.
2. Tonify heart and spleen.

Medicinal Uses:

1. Insomnia, palpitations, dizziness, forgetfulness, and amnesia.
2. Postpartum weakness, and debility.
3. Deficiency of qi and blood.

Contraindications:

1. Persons with fire symptoms.
2. Persons with damp/phlegm symptoms.

Lonicera

(*Jin yin huan*, Honeysuckle, Lonicerae Flos)

Part Used: flower.

Essence and Flavor: sweet, and cold.

Channels Entered: lung, stomach, and large intestine.

Function:

1. Clear heat, and resolve toxin.

2. Antibacterial.
3. Antipyretic, and antiinflammatory.

Medicinal:

1. Common cold caused by wind and heat.
2. Febrile diseases with high fever, and thirst.
3. Upper respiratory tract.
4. Boils, and furuncles.
5. Enteritis, and dysentery.
6. Urinary tract infection.

Contraindications: persons with deficiency and cold symptoms.

Pharmaceutical Action:

1. Antibacterial (broad spectrum)--inhibit the growth of Staph. aureus, hemolytic streptococcus, B. dysenteriae, B. typhi, meningococcus, pneumococcus, virus, etc.
2. Decreases the absorption of cholesterol from the intestine in experimental rabbits.
3. Reduce blood pressure--used in combination with chrysanthemum flower for high blood pressure and arteriosclerosis.
4. Prevention of gastric ulcer (mild action).
5. The injection form can be used for the treatment of acute tonsillitis.

Lotus Seed

(*Shi lian zi*, Nelumbonis Semen)

Part Used: seed.

Essence and Flavor: sweet, astringent, and neutral.

Channels Entered: spleen, and kidney.

Function:

1. Tonify the spleen, and stop diarrhea.
2. Tonify the kidney, and arrest seminal emission.
3. Sedative.

Medicinal Uses:

1. Chronic diarrhea, and lack of appetite.
2. Spontaneous seminal emission, and leukorrhea.
3. Insomnia, and palpitation.

Contraindications: persons with constipation, and abdominal distention.

Magnolia

(*Hou pu*, Magnoliae Officinalis Cortex)

Part Used: bark.

Essence and Flavor: pungent, bitter and warm.

Channels Entered: spleen, stomach, lung, and large intestine.

Function:

1. Promote the flow of vital energy, and relieve food stagnation in the stomach.
2. Invigorate the function of the spleen by drying up dampness.
3. Reverse the upward flow of qi of the lung to relieve asthma,

Medicinal Uses:

1. Gastralgia, and abdominal distention.
2. Vomiting, and nausea due to dyspepsia.
3. Cough and asthma with profuse phlegm.
4. Diarrhea.

Contraindications: pregnant women and persons with spleen and stomach deficiency.

Ma-huang

(*Ma huang*, Ephedra, Mormon tea,
yellow hemp, Ephedrae Herba)

Parts Used: twigs and stems.

Essence and Flavor: pungent, bitter, and warm.

Channels Entered: lung, and urinary bladder.

Function:

1. Diaphoretic.
2. Antiasthmatic.
3. Diuretic, and to regulate water metabolism.

Medicinal Uses:

1. Common cold due to wind and cold.
2. Cough, and asthma.
3. Acute nephritic edema.
4. Ostealgia, and arthralgia.

Contraindications: persons with insomnia, spontaneous sweating, high blood pressure, cardiac asthma, and weak stomach.

Ophiopogon

(*Mai men dong,* Ophiopogonis Tuber)

Part Used: root.

Essence and Flavor: sweet, slightly bitter, and cold.

Channels Entered: heart, lung, and stomach.

Function:

1. Replenishes vital essence.
2. Promotes secretion of body fluids.
3. Nourishes stomach and heart.
4. Soothes lungs.

Medicinal Uses:

1. Thirst, and dry throat.
2. Dry stools due to stomach yin xu.
3. Dry cough with thin or bloody sputum.
4. Palpitations, insomnia, fear, and fullness.

Contraindications: diarrhea due to coldness, stomach, and spleen *yang xu*.

Pangolin

(*Chuan shan jia*, Manitis Squama)

Part Used: scales.

Essence and Flavor: salty, and slightly cold.

Channel Entered: liver and stomach.

Functions:

1. Emmenagogue and galactagogue (aids menstrual flow and lactation).
2. Reduces inflammation and blood stasis.
3. Dispels pus.
4. Hemostatic (external use only).

Medicinal Use:

1. Amenorrhea, and deficiency of lactation.
2. Tumors, and scrofula.
3. Acute purulent inflammation and abscess.
4. External trauma.

Contraindications: persons with deficiency of qi and blood symptoms.

Pharmaceutical Action: increases the count of WBC.

Phellodendron

(*Huang-bo*, Phellodendri Cortex)

Part Used: root.

Essence and Flavor: bitter, and cold.

Channels Entered: kidney, urinary bladder, and large intestine.

Function:

1. Eliminate heat and dampness.
2. Sedate fire, and detoxify.
3. Antibacterial.
4. Reduce heat caused by deficiency of vital essence.

Medicinal Uses:

1. Diarrhea, jaundice, leukorrhea, dysentery, and acute UTI.
2. Abscess, eczema, boils, and furuncles.
3. Chronic tidal fever with night sweats and seminal emissions.

Contraindications: persons with diarrhea or a weak stomach.

Pinellia

(*Ban xia*, Pinelliae Tuber)

Part Used: tuber.

Essence and Flavor: pungent, warm, and toxic.

Channels Entered: lung, spleen, and stomach.

Function:

1. Eliminate phlegm and dampness.
2. Reverse the flow of qi.
3. Disperse lumps and hardenings.
4. Harmonize stomach.
5. Control vomiting.

Medicinal Uses:

1. Cough with profuse thin phlegm caused by dampness.
2. Nausea, vomiting, and morning sickness.
3. Stuffiness in the chest, scrofula, globus hystericus, and deep rooted ulcer.

Contraindications: pregnant women (in later stages), any kind of blood disorder, intestinal fluids, and shao yang and tai yin stages of disease.

Pinellia

(*Ban xia*, Half Summer, Pinellia Tuber)

Part Used: root.

Essence and Flavor: acrid, warm, and poisonous.

Channels Entered: spleen, and stomach.

Functions:

1. Dry dampness.
2. Transform phlegm.
3. Cause rebellious qi to descend.
4. Harmonize the stomach.
5. Dissipate nodules.

Indications: goiter, scrofula, cold phlegm in the lungs, and vomiting.

Contraindications: deficient yin, all cases of bleeding, and excess heat conditions.

Platycodon

(*Jie geng*, Platycodi Radix)

Part Used: root.

Essence and Flavor: bitter, pungent, and neutral.

Channel Entered: lung.

Functions:

1. Ventilate and smooth the lung.
2. Disperse cold, and resolve phlegm due to wind cold or wind heat.
3. Eliminate pus.

Medicinal Uses:

1. Cough with profuse phlegm due to infection in the respiratory tract.
2. Throat inflammation.
3. Pulmonary abscess.

Contraindications: persons with tuberculosis.

Polyporus

(*Zhu ling*, Polyporus)

Part Used: sclerotium of fungus.

Essence and Flavor: sweet, light flavor, and neutral.

Channels Entered: kidney, and urinary bladder.

Function:

1. Diuretic; promote dieresis, and eliminate dampness.
2. Dispel heat.

Medicinal Uses:

1. Edema, and dysuria.
2. Urinary disturbances with turbid discharge.
3. Morbid leukorrhea.

Contraindications: persons with no circulation of water, and those with dampness in the body.

Pueraria Flower

(*Ge hua*, Puerariae Flos)

Part Used: flower.

Essence and Flavor: sweet, and cool.

Channel Entered: stomach.

Function:

1. Relieve alcoholic poisoning.
2. Dispel heat in the stomach.

Medicinal Uses:

1. Thirst.
2. High fever.
3. Abdominal fullness.
4. Nausea and vomiting due to alcohol poisoning.
5. Intestinal hemorrhage.

Pueraria

(*Go Gen*, Puerariae Radix)

Part Used: root (in Pueraria Combination).

Essence and Flavor: sweet, pungent, and cool.

Channels Entered: spleen. and stomach.

Function:

1. Diaphoretic.
2. Relieve pain in the neck and back.
3. Relieve thirst due to febrile conditions.
4. Promote eruptions in measles.
5. Wind-cold or wind-heat invasion.
6. Antihypertensive.

Medicinal Uses:

1. Common cold with discomfort and pain in the neck and back.
2. Febrile disease and diabetes.
3. Hypertension, headache, and coronary heart disease.
4. Measles.

Contraindications: persons with excessive sweating and coldness in the stomach.

Rhubarb

(*Da huang*, Rhei Rhizoma)

Part Used: rhizoma.

Essence and Flavor: bitter, and cold.

Channels Entered: spleen, stomach, large intestine, pericardium, and liver.

Functions:

1. Disperses dryness.
2. Purges and detoxifies.
3. Relieves stagnant blood and heat.
4. Cleans stomach.

Medicinal Uses:

1. Abdominal pain.
2. Delirium.

3. Thirst.
4. Constipation.
5. Hypertension.

Contraindication: pregnancy.

Safflower

(Carthamus, *Hong hua*, Carthami Tinctorius)

Part Used: flower.

Essence and Flavor: pungent, and warm.

Channels Entered: liver, and heart.

Function:

1. Invigorate the circulation of the blood, and remove blood stasis.
2. Analgesic.

Medicinal Uses:

1. Amenorrhea, dysmenorrhea, abdominal pain, and tumors.
2. Traumatic injury.
3. Hepatomegaly, and splenomegaly.

Contraindication: pregnant women, and women with menorrhagia.

Pharmaceutical Action:

1. Excitatory action on the uterus--produces tonic or rhythmic contractions. Large dosages can increase the autonomic contraction rate, even to the degree of spasms. This action is even obvious in a pregnant uterus. It is also fast acting and endures long.
2. Action on the circulatory system:
   a. Constriction of the renal blood vessels to decrease the blood flow to the kidney.
   b. Dilation of the coronary artery.
   c. Lower blood pressure, and useful over a long time.
3. Excitatory action on the smooth muscle of the intestines, blood vessels, and bronchi.

4. Small dosages have excitatory action on the heart (mild degree), large dosages have inhibitory action.
5. Protection from ischemic and anoxic brain injury, and effective for ischemic cerebral diseases.
6. Lowers cholesterol, total lipids, and triglycerides.
7. Oral intake of safflower oil, 1 gm/kg/day, can be used in hypercholesteremia.

Carthamine:

1. Used in dye industry for the coloring of drugs and candies.

Smilax

(*Tu fu ling*,
Smooth Greenbrier, Smilacis Glabrae Rhizoma)

Part Used: rhizoma.

Essence and Flavor: sweet to taste, and neutral.

Channels Entered: liver, and stomach.

Function:

1. Detoxicant.
2. Dispel dampness (antiarthritic).

Medicinal Uses:

1. Infection of the urinary system, syphilis, furuncles, and carbuncles.
2. Rheumatoid arthritis.

Contraindications: persons with deficiency of yin (vital essence) of liver and kidney.

Others: *Tu fu ling* can neutralize mercury poisoning. It is excellent for syphilis, especially the secondary and tertiary stages.

Stephania

(*Fang chi*, Aristolochiae Fangchi Radix)

Part Used: root.

Essence and Flavor: pungent, bitter, and cold.

Channels Entered: lung, spleen, urinary bladder, and kidney.

Function:

1. Antirheumatic--relieves pain due to wind and dampness.
2. Diuretic--relieves water retention due to spleen and kidney *yang xu*.

Medicinal Uses:

1. Rheumatic arthritis.
2. Edema, and oliguria.

Contraindications: persons with accumulation of dampness.

Tribulus

(*Ji li*, Tribuli Fructus)

Part Used: fruit.

Essence and Flavor: pungent, bitter, neutral, mild, and warm.

Channels Entered: liver, and kidney.

Function:

1. Restore the activity of the vital function (yang) of the liver.
2. Dispel wind, and clear the eyes.

Medicinal Uses:

1. Hypertensive headache, and dizziness.
2. Fullness of the chest.
3. Mastitis, and acute conjunctivitis.

Contraindications: pregnant women, and persons with qi and blood deficiency.

Pharmaceutical Action:

1. Lowers blood pressure.
2. Diuretic--due to the presence of potassium ion.
3. Counteract the activity of acetylcholine.
4. Antibacterial--against Staph. aureus, E. coli, etc.
5. Reduction of potassium nitrate may lead to suffocation.

Trichosanthes Root

(*Kua-lou-ken*, *Gau lou gen*, Trichosanthis Radix)

Part Used: root.

Essence and Flavor: slightly sweet/bitter, sour, and cold.

Channels Entered: lung, and stomach.

Function:

1. Clear internal heat, and stimulate the secretion of fluids.
2. Reduce inflammation and dispel pus.

Medicinal Uses:

1. Thirst (as in diabetes).
2. Dry cough, and spitting blood.
3. Inflammation, and abscess.
4. Artificial abortion.

Contraindications: persons with diarrhea, lack of true heat symptoms.

Wheat

(*Fu xiao mai*, Tritici Fructus)

Part Used: light grain.

Essence and Flavor: sweet, and cool.

Channels Entered: heart, and lungs.

Function:

1. Antihydrotic--to stop perspiration caused by qi or yin deficiency.
2. Nourishes the heart, and calms the spirit.

Medicinal Uses:

1. Spontaneous sweating due to deficiency of qi.
2. Night sweats due to deficiency of yin.
3. Irritability, and mental instability.

Contraindications: persons with cold and dampness symptoms.

Zizyphus

(*Suan Zao Ren*, Jujube Seed)

(Zizyphi Spinosi Semen)

Part Used: dried seed.

Essence and Flavor: sweet, sour, and neutral.

Channels Entered: heart, spleen, liver, and gallbladder.

Function:

1. Sedate, tranquilize, and reinforce yin.
2. Anhidrotic (stops perspiration).
3. Nourish the liver.

Medicinal Uses:

1. Insomnia, and palpitations.
2. Night sweats, and spontaneous perspiration.
3. Lower blood pressure.
4. Diaphoresis due to deficiency.

Contraindication: evil fire in the body.

Zizyphus

(*Da zao*, Jujube, Zizyphi Fructus)

Part Used: fruit.

Essence and Flavor: sweet, and warm.

Channel Entered: spleen.

Function:

1. Supplements and toxifies the spleen and stomach, and moistens heart and lungs.
2. Nourishes and pacifies spirit.
3. Smoothes herbal action.
4. Harmonizes all drugs.

Medicinal Uses:

1. Antiallergic effect.
2. Antiulcer effect.

SINGLE HERB LIST

Achyranthes	*Achyranthis Radix*	*Niu xi*
Aconite (processed)	*Aconiti Carmichaelii Praeparata Radix*	*Fu zi*
Acorus	*Acori Rhizoma*	*Chang pu*
Akebia	*Akebiae Caulis*	*Mu tong*
Alisma	*Alismatis Rhizoma*	*Ze xie*
Anemarrhena	*Anemarrhenae Rhizoma*	*Zhi mu*
Angelica	*Angelicae Dahuricae Radix*	*Bai zhi*
Apricot Seed	*Armeniacae Semen*	*Xing ren*
Areca Seed	*Arecae Semen*	*Bing lang zi*
Arisaema	*Arisaematis Rhizoma*	*Tian nan xing*
Artemisia	*Artemisiae Argyi Folium*	*Ai ye*
Asarum	*Asari Herba Cum Radice*	*Xi xin*
Asparagus	*Asparagi Radix*	*Tian men dong*
Astragalus	*Astragali Radix*	*Huang qi*
Atractylodes (red)	*Atractylodis Lanceae Rhizoma*	*Cang zhu*
Atractylodes (white)	*Atractylodis Rhizoma*	*Bai zhu*
Bamboo (shavings)	*Bambusae Caulis et Taeniis*	*Zhu ru*
Benincasa	*Benincasae Semen*	*Dong gua zi*
Biota	*Biotae Semen*	*Bo zi ren*
Blue Citrus	*Citri Immaturi Pericarpium*	*Qing pi*
Bupleurum	*Bupleuri Radix*	*Chai hu*
Capillaris	*Artemisiae Capillaris Herba*	*Yin chen hao*
Carthamus	*Carthami Flos*	*Hong hua*

Chaenomeles	*Chaenomelis Fructus*	*Mu gua*
Cherry bark	*Pruni Cortex*	*Yin pi*
Chih-ko	*Aurantii Fructus*	*Zhi ko*
Chih-shih	*Aurantii Fructus Immaturus*	*Zhi shi*
Chiang-huo	*Notopterygii Rhizoma*	*Qiang huo*
Cimicifuga	*Cimicifugae Rhizoma*	*Sheng ma*
Cinnabar	*Cinnabaris*	*Zhu sha*
Cinnamon Bark	*Cinnamomi Cortex*	*Gui pi*
Cinnamon Twigs	*Cinnamomi Ramulus*	*Gui zhi*
Citrus (dried)	*Citri Leiocarpae Exocarpium*	*Chen-pi*
Clematis	*Clematidis Radix*	*Wei ling xian*
Cnidium	*Cnidii Rhizoma (Ligustici Rhizoma)*	*Chuan xiong*
Coix	*Coicis Semen*	*Yi yi ren*
Coptis	*Coptidis Rhizoma*	*Huang lian*
Cornus	*Corni Fructus*	*Shan zhu yu*
Croton	*Semen Crotonis*	*Ba dou*
Cyperus	*Cyperi Rhizoma*	*Xiang fu zi*
Dendrobium	*Dendrobii Caulis*	*Shi hu*
Dioscorea	*Dioscorea Batatis Rhizoma*	*Shan yao*
Dragon Bone	*Draconis Os*	*Long gu*
Eriobotrya	*Eriobotryae Folium*	*Pi pa ye*
Evodia	*Evodiae Fructus*	*Wu zhu yu*
Flava Wax	*Cera Flava*	*Huang la*
Forsythia	*Forsythiae Fructus*	*Lian qiao*
Fritillaria	*Fritillariae Bulbus*	*Bei mu*
Gadfly	*Tabanus*	*Meng chung*
Gambir	*Uncariae Ramulus et Uncus*	*Gou teng*
Gardenia	*Gardeniae Fructus*	*Zhi zi*
Gelatin	*Asini Gelatinum*	*A jiao*
Gentiana	*Gentianae Scabrae Radix*	*Long dan*
Ginger (fresh)	*Zingiberis Rhizoma*	*Sheng jiang*
Ginger (dried)	*Zingiberis Siccatum Rhizoma*	*Gan jiang*
Ginseng	*Ginseng Radix*	*Ren shen*

Gypsum	*Gypsum Fibrosum*	*Shi gao*
Hematite	*Haematitum*	*Dai zhe shi*
Hoelen	*Poria*	*Fu ling*
Ho-shou-wu	*Polygoni Multiflori Radix*	*He shou wo*
Jujube	*Zizyphi Fructus*	*Da zao*
Kaolin	*Halloysitum Rubrum*	*Chi shi zhi*
Laminaria	*Laminariae Thallus*	*Hai dai*
Lard		*Zhu you*
Leech	*Hirudo*	*Shui zhi*
Licorice	*Glycyrrhizae Radix*	*Gan cao*
Lily	*Lilii Bulbus*	*Bai he*
Lindera	*Linderae Radix*	*Wu yao*
Lithospermum	*Lithospermi Radix*	*Zi cao*
Longan	*Longanae Arillus*	*Long yan rou*
Lonicera	*Lonicerae Flos*	*Jin yin hua*
Lotus Seed	*Nelumbonis Semen*	*Lian zi*
Lycium Bark	*Lycii Radicis Cortex*	*Di gu pi*
Magnolia Bark	*Magnoliae Officinalis Cortex*	*Hou pu*
Magnolia Flower	*Magnoliae Liliflorae Flos*	*Xin yi*
Ma-huang	*Ephedrae Herba*	*Ma huang*
Mentha	*Menthae Herba*	*Bo he*
Mirabilitum	*Natrium Sulfuricum*	*Mang xiao*
Morus Bark	*Mori Radicis Cortex*	*Sang bai pi*
Moutan	*Moutan Radicis Cortex*	*Mu dan pi*
Ophiopogon	*Ophiopogonis Tuber*	*Mai men tong*
Oryza	*Oryza Semen*	*Jing mi*
Oyster Shell	*Ostreae Testa*	*Mu li*
Pangolin	*Mantis Squama*	*Chuan shan jia*
Peony	*Paeoniae Radix*	*Shao yao*
Perilla	*Perillae*	*Zi su*
Perilla Leaves	*Perillae Folium*	*Zi su ye*
Persica	*Persicae Semen*	*Tao ren*
Phellodendron	*Phellodendri Cortex*	*Huang bo*
Pinellia	*Pinellia Tuber*	*Ban xia*

Plantago	*Plantaginis Semen*	*Che qian zi*
Platycodon	*Platycodi Radix*	*Jie geng*
Polygala	*Polygalae Radix*	*Yuan zhi*
Polyporus	*Polyporus*	*Zhu ling*
Pueraria	*Pueriae Radix*	*Ge gen*
Rehmannia (cooked)	*Rehmanniae Radix*	*Shu di huang*
Rehmannia (raw)	*Rehmanniae Radix*	*Sheng di huang*
Rhubarb	*Rhei Rhizoma*	*Da huang*
Salvia	*Salviae Miltiorrhziae Radix*	*Dan shen*
Saussurea	*Saussureae Radix*	*Mu xiang*
Schizandra	*Schizandrae Fructus*	*Wu wei zi*
Schizonepeta	*Schizonepetae Herba*	*Jing jie*
Scirpus	*Sparganii Rhizoma*	*San ling*
Scrophularia	*Scrophulariae Radix*	*Xuan shen*
Scute	*Scutellariae Radix*	*Huang qin*
Seaweed	*Sargassum*	*Hai zao*
Sesame Oil	*Oleum Sesami*	*Hu ma you*
Siler	*Ledebouriellae Radix*	*Fang feng*
Smilax	*Smilacis Glabrae Rhizoma*	*Tu fu ling*
Stephania	*Aristolochiae Fangchi Radix*	*Fang chi*
Talc	*Talcum and Kaolinum*	*Hua shi*
Tang-kuei	*Angelicae Radix*	*Dang gui*
Terminalia	*Chebulae Fructus*	*Ke zi*
Trapa	*Trapae Fructus*	*Ling jiao*
Tribulus	*Tribuli Fructus*	*Ji li*
Trichosanthes Root	*Trichosanthis Radix*	*Gua lou gen*
Trichosanthes Seed	*Trichosanthis Semen*	*Gua lou ren*
Tu-huo	*Angelicae Tuhuo Radix*	*Du huo*
Wheat	*Tritici Fructus*	*Fu xiao mai*
Wisteria	*Wisteria Galla*	*Teng Liu*
Zedoaria	*Zedoariae Rhizoma*	*E zhu*
Zizyphus	*Zizyphi Spinosi Semen*	*Suan zao ren*

GENERAL INDEX

A

C

D

E

F

I

J

K

L

M

P

R

S

T

U

INDEX OF FORMULAS

A

B

C

R

S

T

V

W

Z

REFERENCES

1. Hsu, Hong-Yen. *Oriental Materia Medica: A Concise Guide*. OHAI, Long Beach, Ca. 1986.
2. Hsu, Hong-Yen. An Outline of Oriental Materia Medica. *Bulletin of the Oriental Healing Arts Institute of U.S.A.* Long Beach, Ca. 1984
3. Hsu, Hong-Yen, and Wang, Su-Yen (translators). *Chin Kuei Yao Lueh*. OHAI, Long Beach, Ca. 1983.
4. Hsu, Hong-Yen, and Haueter, Judith (ed.). *Chinese Herbal Science*. OHAI, Long Beach, Ca. 1982.
5. Hsu, Hong-Yen, and Easer, Douglas H. *For Women Only: Chinese Herbal Formulas*. OHAI, Long Beach, Ca. 1982.
6. Hsu, Hong-Yen. *Natural Healing with Chinese Herbs*. OHAI, Long Beach, Ca. 1982.
7. Hsu, Hong-Yen, and Peacher, William (ed.). *Shang Han Lun*. OHAI, Long Beach, Ca. 1981.
8. Hsu, Hong-Yen, and Hsu, Chau Shin. *Commonly Used Chinese Herb Formulas*. OHAI, Long Beach, Ca. 1980.
9. Hsu, Hong-Yen. *How to Treat Yourself with Chinese Herbs*. OHAI, Long Beach, Ca. 1980.
10. Moore, James Michael. *A Study of the Six Stages of Disease and The Chinese Medical Classics Shang Han Lun and Chin Kuei Yao Lueh*. Dissertation submitted to the Southwest Acupuncture College), Santa Fe, N.M. 1988.
11. Moore, James Michael. Class Notes, Classical Chinese Medical Methods 301-302. Southwest Acupuncture College, Santa Fe, N.M. 1986-87.